Newton's
MADNESS

HAROLD L. KLAWANS, M.D.

Newton's

Further Tales of Clinical Neurology

MADNESS

HarperPerennial
A Division of HarperCollins*Publishers*

Grateful acknowledgment is made to the following for permission to quote copyrighted material:

From "I Get a Kick Out of You," by Cole Porter. © 1934 (renewed). Warner Bros. Inc. All Rights Reser▪ Used by Permission.

A hardcover edition of this book was published in 1990 by Harper & Row, Publishers, Inc.

First HarperPerennial edition published 1991.

To my patients

=Contents=

=== Acknowledgments ===

My job description as an academic neurologist includes three facets: research, teaching, and patient care. All three compete for my time and my imagination. Most academicians use up most, if not all, of their inspiration on their research. Over the years I have dedicated much of mine to teaching. One of the methods I employ in teaching is the use of history and historical vignettes to amplify and/or emphasize points that would otherwise be passed over all too easily. These have been collected from numerous sources over the years in an endless process. In this book as in *Toscanini's Fumble,* I have put together a number of these tales in the types of clinical settings in which I would tell them to my residents. Much of the material therefore in a sense is not "original." History never can be. I have added a note at the end of each chapter listing the most important sources.

I wish to thank Rick Kot for his incisive and thoughtful editing of the final manuscript.

Newton's
MADNESS

Although all the case studies featured in this book are true, in many instances the names and identifying characteristics of contemporary subjects have been changed to protect the privacy of those individuals.

═Prologue═

I have said it before, but a teacher who hesitates to repeat, shrinks from his most important duty, and a learner who dislikes to hear the same thing twice over lacks his most essential acquisition.
—William R. Gowers (1845–1915), noted English neurologist

Do you know my name?'' I asked the patient. I did not expect Mr. Hayes to recall my name. He had been my patient for only a few days. We had met only a couple of times. And he had severe memory difficulties that we thought would turn out to be due to Alzheimer's disease.

He looked at me quizzically, as if he was trying to summon whatever ability to recall names that remained functioning. ''Would it help me if I did?'' he finally replied.

''No,'' I admitted, ''probably not.''

''What year is it?'' the resident asked him.

''Nineteen forty-five,'' he replied.

''He's wiped out,'' the resident went on, addressing this remark to me, not to Mr. Hayes. ''Where are you?'' he asked the patient.

''At home.''

''What am I doing here?''

That was probably almost as good a question as the one Mr. Hayes had asked me. But the patient's growing anger was becoming apparent, for the resident seemed to be attacking whatever dignity he had left. The resident did not want to shame him; he was merely demonstrating the degree of the dementia. Not that it needed to be publicly exposed—we all knew that it was not 1945.

''You a Cub fan?'' I interrupted.

''You bet.''

''Nineteen forty-five. Who's our first baseman?''

''Phil Cavaretta.''

He was right; Phil Cavaretta had played first base for the '45 Cubs. In no time at all, he gave me the entire starting lineup of the pennant-winning

1945 Cubs. We didn't attempt to name the pitching staff, not because he couldn't have done it, but because I could only remember Hank Borowy.

"Thank you, Doctor Klawans," he said as I left his bedside.

My interaction with Frank Hayes, like most of the vignettes I have gathered during my career as a neurologist, reminds me of classical Greek tragedy. The comparison is not intended to reflect the serious and often even tragic nature of the diseases that make up a neurologist's life and, more significantly, the lives of his patients. The analogy between severe neurologic disease and a tragic flaw is not all that poetic. The similarity that impresses me, rather, is a structural one. When a patient first comes to see me, his or her story has already begun. Like a classic tragedy, our interaction opens *in medias res,* in the midst of things, with the events of the past played out selectively and rapidly before my eyes. And then when our brief encounter is over, the patient is left to live his or her life. That life may be altered in some way by our interaction. But whether it is or it isn't, the interaction of the patient and the disease that antedated our meeting inevitably extends beyond it.

Oedipus Rex starts in the midst of the life of King Oedipus. The tragedy has already been set into motion. The disease exists. Oedipus's self-discovery, his self-diagnosis, and his self-induced therapeutic resolution are all that are required to complete the play. And once they have occurred, Oedipus is left, altered, to live out his life.

Too dramatic? Too melodramatic? Perhaps. But perhaps it is that very concept of structure that forces me to care what happens to my patients outside of the confines of my office. And to try to write about them as they live out their lives.

I teach at Rush Medical College, named after Benjamin Rush, signer of the Declaration of Independence and the most renowned physician of the early decades of the United States. Today physicians are trained to be scientists. No one today could possibly accuse Benjamin Rush of having been a scientist. He had no concept of the scientific method. When a yellow fever epidemic struck Philadelphia, Rush responded. He went from bedside to bedside, working twenty hours a day. Patients were dying right and left. There had to be something he could do to help them.

There were purgatives and bloodletting.

Rush bled his patients to restore a better balance.

More died.

He bled them even more.

Even more died.

He hurried from bedside to bedside, tirelessly bleeding patients wherever he went, the beloved Benjamin Rush, yet he may have, by his treatments, killed almost as many of his patients as the yellow fever did. He was a caring physician, but he was not a scientist. And he had been wrong—dead wrong.

Today, we ridicule Rush's foolish theories of disease and dangerous forms of treatment. Rush was not a scientist and made no pretense of being one. He was a physician. Today physicians are scientists. We know science and the scientific method. And in science the one fault is to be wrong. We must make the right diagnosis and then embark on the correct course of therapy. Not because of the threat of a malpractice suit, but because of the fear of being wrong.

It is that fear that leads physicians to rely more on scientific data than on their patients.

Laboratory results, not history.

X rays, not the physical examination.

Logic, not insight.

And never intuition.

And along the way, understanding and caring have gotten lost. These were traits that Rush never lost. They were the tools of his profession.

When Benjamin Rush and his bloodletting were attacked as harmful, it was not the other bloodletters who defended him, but his patients and their families. He could not have hurt them, they believed, because he cared about them. If more of his patients died than did those who went to other physicians, it was not, in the public eye, Benjamin Rush's fault.

We must never forget what all doctors used to know. Today, we teach our students at the bedside of our patients, yet half often ignore the patients themselves. We sometimes forget to listen to what the patients are saying. And often fail to hear. The needs of patients are not identical to the needs of their physicians. The needs are not mutually exclusive, but they are different. The patient needs to be well again, to be whole. That is also what the physician would like to see happen, although it may not in fact be possible. And even if it is possible, one step must come first: the diagnosis.

The doctor is stuck with that fact of life. And of death. Although the patient at some level understands this, his priorities must be different. "Get me well, Doc," is his request, not, "Find out what precise disease I have."

Doctors no longer take apprenticeships. We no longer train by sitting at the side of a sick patient with our mentor waiting out the "crisis" of a disease—that moment that is the turning point and determines the prognosis: recovery or death.

That method was dramatic in its way, and it was supportive. But more than that, it was caring.

The role of the physician today is somehow to strike the needed balance between science and empathy.

We must never forget what all doctors used to know. Today we teach at the bedside. We must also listen, and hear, and reach out to help.

So the next day on rounds, after we went over all the results of Mr. Hayes's various blood tests and looked at his CAT scan and decided whether to perform a spinal tap, I did not ask him my name or the date. Instead, I asked him about Gabby Harnett and the pennant-winning 1938 Cubs. Phil Cavaretta, he recalled, had played in the outfield then.

This is the second book of clinical stories that I have written. The first one is *Toscanini's Fumble*. In both of these books I have adapted vignettes that I had been collecting and using in my clinical teaching of medical students and residents for many years. Incorporating them into these books primarily involved selecting the right tales and restructuring them to work at a different level—that of the interested general reader. But it is basically the same process of telling the stories in order to teach. And teaching is teaching.

Or is it? In teaching medicine, repetition is not only valid, it is a necessary evil. Important concepts must not just be learned, they have to be overlearned—so overlearned that they are recalled immediately at three in the morning when decisions have to be made at the bedside of a critically ill patient. Most of the readers of this book will never be involved in such a decision-making process. Still, the facts that I present are complex and not easy to learn or retain. And since each story should be able to be read on its own, some degree of repetition is at times needed.

I am supposed to be a scientist, not a mystic. Yet in the past doctors were a little bit of both. In physics it is well accepted that the mere act of observing an experiment influences the result. The same is also true in medical experiments. That is why we need to do double-blind studies in which neither the physician nor the patient knows which patient is receiving the active medication and which the placebo.

Observation influences outcome.

Does merely making the diagnosis change the prognosis? We all know of patients who have gone along struggling with some unknown malady for years, are finally given some diagnosis, and die in days. Is this merely coincidence? Or would some of my patients have done better if I hadn't made my diagnosis? And if so, which ones?

And then the mystic in me raises his head. If the diagnosis had never been made, might not the disease have just disappeared? There is no scientific evidence of this. By definition there can't be. I wish I could always be sure that my mystical fears were only that.

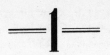

My Mother's Best Friend

I know I am seated, my hands on my knees, because of the pressure against my rump, against the soles of my feet, against the palms of my hands, against my knees. Against my palms the pressure is of my knees, against my knees of my palms, but what is it that presses against my rump, against the soles of my feet? I don't know. My spine is not supported. I mention these details to make sure I am not lying on my back, my legs raised and bent, my eyes closed. It is well to establish the position of the body from the outset, before passing on to more important matters.

—Samuel Beckett, *The Unnamable*

It's very hard to live a productive life when a piece of your brain is missing. And that's what a stroke is, a hole in the brain.

—John P. Conomy, M.D.,
Chairman of Neurology
Cleveland Clinic

Betty was not my aunt, but I grew up thinking she was and calling her Aunt Betty. She and "Uncle George" lived next door to us in an apartment building on the South Side of Chicago. She and my mother did everything together from their morning cup of coffee to grocery shopping to volunteer work with various charities. They were inseparable. It was not until I was ten or twelve that I fully realized that Betty was not a relation at all. It was then that I realized that Aunt Betty and Uncle George never were at "family" functions unless those parties or dinners were at our house.

If my parents were out of town, I stayed with Aunt Betty. If for some reason my Mom couldn't be home to give me lunch, I ate at Aunt Betty's.

Aunt Betty and Uncle George drove my mother to the hospital when she went into labor with me, a tale I was told annually on my birthday by Uncle George until his Alzheimer's disease wiped out that memory for him.

Aunt Betty was from Atlanta. She hadn't gone to college but to a "finishing school." Yet whenever I went over to her place, she would be reading a book—except on Saturday afternoon, when she did her ironing and listened to the broadcast of the Metropolitan Opera. She might not have been able to tell me the significance of the musical development of Verdi's *Luisa Miller* but she could tell after a few bars which soprano was singing and why that soprano was or wasn't living up to her expectations. She was also quick to remind me whenever *I* didn't live up to her expectations—almost as quick as my mother. It was no wonder that they were such close friends.

In 1974, when I was thirty-seven, I began practicing neurology at Michael Reese Hospital—the hospital where I was born. I had been there about six months when my mother called me one morning and told me that Aunt Betty had a stroke. I knew what was to follow before it was said: I was expected to be her doctor. Aunt Betty was on her way to the hospital to be my patient.

"I'm sure you can help her," my mother said. "Most people with strokes get better, and you're the best neurologist in town. You'll get her better."

It was not a question or a command. It was a statement of my mother's expectations. If I was a good neurologist, I could help Aunt Betty.

I said goodbye and took a deep breath. Back in 1974, there was no effective way to treat most strokes, and even today, such treatment is still in its infancy. At that time, care of a stroke patient consisted primarily of doing whatever could be done to allow the patient to heal himself or herself and trying to prevent the next stroke. Thank God, my mother was right. Patients who had strokes did improve. Aunt Betty would get better.

I started my afternoon rounds at one o'clock sharp. The resident told me that there were two new patients to be seen. One was Mrs. Betty Goodman, the other a man named Vartan Essegian. According to the resident, they had both had strokes. I could tell by the sound of his voice that he'd found neither patient to be exciting, just two run-of-the-mill strokes. At Michael Reese, we saw eight to ten patients with strokes each week. Two more were no big deal to him.

He couldn't have been more wrong.

We started by seeing Mr. Essegian, which I would have suggested in any case. Not to delay my trial by fire or because I didn't want to slight a man named after the saint who converted Armenia to Christianity. I was already certain that Betty had a stroke; my mother had told me that much. As to Mr. Essegian's condition, I had the opinion of a resident who had been studying neurology with me for only three years. My mother had been my mother all my life.

The resident, Paul McAnany, took us—two other neurology residents, one internal medicine resident, and four medical students—to see Vartan Essegian. Mr. Essegian's history was straightforward enough. He'd been well when he went to bed. He'd gotten up to go to the bathroom sometime during the night, the exact time we didn't know. His wife had found him at about five in the morning lying on the bathroom floor. He could neither speak nor move his right side. She called an ambulance, knowing he'd had a stroke. *She probably studied with my mother,* I thought to myself.

Mrs. Essegian was right. Her husband, Vartan, had had a stroke, and as I examined him, I saw a number of neurologic problems that were due to his stroke:

1. He could not speak or understand language—a global or total aphasia.
2. He could not move his right arm, his right leg, or the lower part of his right face—a right hemiplegia.
3. His eyes tended to look to the left.

It was time to do some teaching, and teaching is what I did. I even pulled out all the aphorisms I'd been taught as a young resident. Anything to put off the inevitable.

Every stroke results from a region of damaged brain. In each stroke, this damage has come about because of some disorder in which the blood vessels that supply blood to the brain are no longer doing their job adequately. That is the definition of a stroke; but there are a number of ways in which the blood vessels can produce such injuries. So I started with a discussion of the types of stroke:

1. Hemorrhage
2. Embolus
3. Thrombosis or infarction

I made the students define each of these phenomena.

A hemorrhage is a site of fresh bleeding within the substance of the brain. It starts when a small blood vessel—an artery bringing needed oxygen and nutrients to the brain—ruptures and spews blood into the brain. Barring unusual medical conditions, such hemorrhages happen only in patients with high blood pressure.

Did Vartan Essegian have high blood pressure? No.

Such hemorrhages always show up on CAT scans. Did Vartan Essegian's CAT scan show a hemorrhage? No.

So much for a hemorrhage. On to embolus.

An embolus is a blood clot that forms in one place in the body and then breaks off and travels to another place. The commonest site for the formation of emboli is the deep veins of the legs, in a condition known as thrombophlebitis, inflammation of the veins with the formation of thrombi (blood clots). If a thrombus becomes dislodged from the leg, it doesn't go to the brain, but passes through the heart and becomes lodged in the lungs as a pulmonary embolus.

So where do cerebral or brain emboli originate? In the heart. And when they break off they go directly from the heart to the brain.

Why do blood clots form in the heart? Recent heart attacks are one cause.

Was there any evidence that Vartan Essegian had a recent heart attack? No.

The other condition that can cause the formation of blood clots in the heart is heart disease involving dilated chambers and abnormal heart rhythms.

Mr. Essegian's heart was of normal size, and we found no evidence of abnormal rhythms.

There was no reason for a thrombus to form in Mr. Essegian's heart. Without a thrombus, there cannot be an embolus.

So much for an embolus. What was left?

Thrombosis. A thrombosis is also a blood clot. A cerebral thrombosis is a blood clot that forms directly within a cerebral artery and blocks that artery, thereby causing a stroke. In clinical usage, the term cerebral thrombosis is a wastebasket term for every stroke that isn't a hemmorhage or an embolus coming from the heart.

As far as we could tell Mr. Essegian had had a thrombosis on the left side of his brain.

How did we know it was on the left side? Because the left side of the brain controls the right side of the body and speech. And Mr. Essegian had a right hemiparesis and aphasia. Ergo, he had had a left-sided stroke.

Why, I asked the group, did the left side of the brain control the right side of the body and the right side of the brain control the left side of the body? None of them knew why.

On to the aphorisms. These had to do with prognosis, our prediction of things to come. Would Mr. Essegian survive? Would he get better? Only a few patients with a single cerebral thrombosis die of their condition. Some do die of complications, however, and it was our job to try to prevent those.

The patients at risk in these cases have either had a heart attack at the same time or have had a massive stroke.

The CAT scan had not shown a big stroke, and there was no evidence of a heart attack. He would not die from his cerebrovascular accident, which we often reduce to the acronym CVA.

Would he get better?

The students were not sure.

The residents were.

Strokes all get better. The part of the brain that is not functioning as a result of the "thrombosis" is far larger than the area in which all the brain cells have actually died. Only those neurons in the center of the stroke can't recover. As the other cells regain their function, the patient improves.

"What will improve?" I asked. "His speech, his strength, or both equally?"

About this, there was no unanimity of opinion among the residents. I let them vote on their answer.

The vote decided on "both equally."

Neurology, unfortunately, is not a democratic process.

"One or the other," I explained.

The region controlling speech and the region controlling movement of the right side of the body are fairly close to each other but are not identical. They are, in fact, different parts of the brain, separated by almost a centimeter of brain tissue. Most strokes, unless they are massive, are not big enough to include both as part of that area in which the brain cells do not recover.

Which area was affected in this case?

It was too early to tell. Whichever one started to recover first would recover best, and I hoped it would be his speech. Even if his right arm and right leg didn't recover, Mr. Essegian would still be able to walk. Everyone with a stroke can learn to walk, for while the leg becomes spastic and doesn't move the way it should, it can support weight and because of this the patient can learn how to walk.

Mr. Essegian was seventy-two. If his speech recovered and we rehabilitated his gait, even if he couldn't use his right arm, life would not be all bad. But without speech, things would be very different.

They all nodded their agreement.

It was time to see Aunt Betty. *It wouldn't be so bad,* I assured myself.
Strokes get better. Nature would run its course. Betty would improve, and
my mother would know I was a good neurologist.

We all walked over to Betty's room. As we made our way, one of the
medical students, a young woman named Barbara Phillips, began to tell
me Betty's history.

Betty had known heart disease.

Known to whom? Not me. How could Aunt Betty have had heart disease
and I not be aware of it? She'd been my aunt for thirty-seven years, I
reminded myself, not my patient.

She had, I was told, rheumatic heart disease with an abnormal heart
and altered heart rhythm. *A large heart and abnormal rhythms. A real
setup for an embolus,* I thought to myself. *Classic, in fact. Just like in
the textbooks.*

When Betty had woken up in the morning and tried to get out of bed,
her left leg gave out. Her husband called my mother, who had made the
diagnosis and the arrangements to admit Betty to Michael Reese under my
care. And I thought only I had the authority to admit patients to my
service.

"What were the clinical findings?" I asked.

"Left hemiplegia," I was told.

Thank God. No aphasia. Aphasia occurs only in strokes of the dominant
(left) hemisphere.

I already felt better.

We discussed the differential diagnosis as we had with Vartan Essegian.
Our conclusion was different.

My Aunt Betty had an embolus—an embolus from a blood clot in the
heart.

We next discussed her prognosis. Unless she had a hemorrhage or a
massive embolus, her prognosis was good. She would certainly live, and
she would get better. Her neurologic function would improve. Nature would
take its course. Recovery.

She would be completely normal mentally: No confusion, no speech
problems. *Normal.*

She might never recover completely, but her right arm was fine. She
could still write. And she'd be able to walk.

I felt a lot better, but the feeling lasted only until I entered her room
and walked to her bedside. It was at that moment that I knew disaster
had struck.

As medical students, we are taught to approach the patient from the
right side, whether it is because the liver is on the right and the spleen is

on the left or because that is how you mount a horse, I really didn't know; tradition seems to be the best explanation.

There is, however, one exception to this rule, an exception I taught myself. If a patient has a left hemiplegia, you approach from the left. Why? Because occasionally patients with left hemiplegia will not be able to direct their attention to anything or anyone to their left. They neglect or are unaware of the left side of their body, and the left side of the world.

The easiest way to detect this condition is to approach them from the left, and so I led everyone to the left side of the bed.

Betty was lying on her back, her head turned to her right. Perhaps the nurses had put her in that position.

Her eyes were turned to the right; it hadn't been the nurses who had done that.

I called her name. "Betty." Not Aunt Betty, but Betty. I was thirty-seven; I'd dropped the "Aunt" long ago—at least two years earlier.

She did not move; did not turn her head or even her eyes.

"Betty," I said again louder, although I knew that her hearing was not the problem.

Again no response.

"Aunt Betty," I said.

"Hal," she replied. "Where are you?"

She was in trouble.

We both were.

She had heard my voice and had recognized it. She was awake, alert, yet had not turned her head or her eyes to look toward me. I was off to her left in what neurologists call the left half of her extrapersonal space. When you call a patient from the left she will look to the left or turn to the left. Unless . . . That was not an unless I wanted to contemplate.

I was standing not two feet from her. Other than through my voice, which came to her as if out of nowhere, I didn't exist.

I turned her head gently so she was facing straight up. Her eyes were still turned to the right.

I lifted her left arm. It was flaccid, loose, with no muscle tone. It was as if her wrinkled skin was all that held the bones together.

I dropped her arm, and it fell back onto the bed like a sack of potatoes. The leg felt the same and fell just the same way.

She had a left hemiplegia—a total left hemiplegia with no muscle tone.

I spoke to her again. Her head never turned toward me, and her eyes continued to look away from me and from the entire crowd gathered to the left of her bed. Her eyes stared off to the right, toward the full half of her world.

We talked on, and it was clear that her speech was normal. There was no aphasia, no memory loss, no confusion. Her mental functions were all normal. It was my Aunt Betty. As bright and clever as ever.

I lifted up her right hand and held it in front of her eyes.

"What is this?"

"My right hand, of course," she remarked with the same intonation she'd always used when she thought I'd done something I shouldn't have or said something foolish.

I let go of her right hand, and she moved it down until it rested on the bed.

I held up her left hand so it was in front of her eyes.

"What is this?" I asked.

"A hand."

"Whose hand?"

She seemed genuinely puzzled.

"Whose hand?" I repeated.

"Your hand," she decided.

I was careful not to drop her hand, for if I had, it would have fallen straight down and struck her in the face. I replaced it carefully on the bed.

"Where are you?"

"Michael Reese Hospital?"

"Why are you here?"

She thought about that one for a while. "To see you." I could tell by her inflection that I had not asked a foolish question. She just didn't know the answer.

"Is anything wrong with you?"

"No."

"How about your left arm? Your left hand?"

"My left hand is fine. How's yours?"

"Mine is also fine," I replied.

There was nothing else to do.

We have a lot of terms for what was wrong with Betty Goodman. Names, theories, classifications, but no treatments.

It was my job to teach my students those names and classifications.

I started with agnosia.

Agnosia means without knowledge.

We all know the parts of our body, where each part is, and what it is doing each and every second of our lives. That awareness belongs to our unconscious knowledge of the world.

When someone approaches a doorway, he or she does not have to check where his head is to be sure it will fit through. Each of us has gotten in and out of a car thousands of times, and rarely, if ever, do we hit our heads on the doorframe of even an unfamiliar car. But a hat is another matter, especially if you don't always wear one. Hats are expendable; they are not part of our unconscious body image.

Body image is integrated in the parietal lobe—the lobe of the brain that begins behind the motor strip (the place where movements are initiated) and extends to the occipital lobe, the back end of the brain, where vision is perceived. The parietal lobe is involved primarily with sensation: the sense of touch, the sense of pressure, the localization of pain to the correct site of the body that is the source of the pain, the localization of temperature sensation, conscious position sense, and unconscious position sense.

All these sensations and others are relayed by parts of the body via the nerves, the nerve tracts in the spinal cord, and the brain stem and eventually end up in the parietal lobe. It is the parietal lobe that integrates physical sensations, and it is through this integration that we are able to discern where we are, where our head is, where our arm is.

And what our body looks like.

When I lifted up Betty's arm, she should have felt me touch her.

Touch sensation.

But she didn't—at least not in a way that reached her consciousness.

She should also have felt it as I lifted her arm. In lifting, touch becomes more than touch, for I was now exerting pressure.

Pressure sensation.

She should have felt that and known precisely where the pressure was being exerted.

She didn't.

She should have felt her arm moving. As I raised her arm, the joints shifted their positions. Joints are loaded with sensory nerves. Normally, if a patient's finger is moved just one or two degrees, the patient can tell you without looking which finger has been moved and both the direction of the movement and its amplitude.

I moved Betty's arm up and across her body.

She had no idea that I had done so.

Then I had held her hand in front of her eyes.

She had seen a hand and she had recognized it as one. Her occipital lobe was receiving the visual input and interpreting it as well as it could, but the parietal lobe had lost its ability to differentiate self from nonself.

She had agnosia, a bad agnosia, involving all forms of sensation, including vision.

She could not recognize part of her own body. That condition is sometimes called autotopagnosia, which means "without knowledge of the topography of self," that is, parts of the body.

And she had a hemiplegia and didn't even know it.

How could she know her left side was paralyzed? She didn't even recognize it. Another specialized word is sometimes used to denote this sort of denial of left hemiplegia: "anosognosia." Before Betty had her stroke, I had disliked all those terms. Now I was beginning to hate them.

And she wouldn't even look to the left. The left half of the world, which is normally integrated in the right parietal lobe, did not exist for her. That's called neglect.

To have all these symptoms simultaneously, and to this degree, meant that virtually all Betty's parietal lobe was not working. She'd had a large stroke—not a massive one, at least not in size. But massive by location.

Unless she started to recover parietal lobe function quickly, she would never walk again.

"Why not?" Barbara Phillips asked.

"If she doesn't know she has an arm and a leg, we can't teach her how to use them. If she doesn't know where her leg is, she'll never be able to walk."

"When will we know if she'll recover?"

I was afraid I already knew.

I looked at the CAT scan. She had suffered a moderate-size stroke just where it had to be, just where I wished it wasn't. The stroke involved the motor strip and much of the parietal lobe.

"Let's give her three or four days," I said, trying to be optimistic. "If she can recognize her arm and leg then and knows what's wrong, she may do fairly well."

Three days later Vartan Essegian started to regain his speech. When he went home three weeks later, he was speaking well enough to be understood and he was walking with a cane.

On the day Vartan started to speak, Betty still did not recognize her left hand and had no idea that she was paralyzed on the left side. She never really recovered. Eventually, she understood she'd had a stroke and would tell me that she was aware of just what was wrong with her. Her left arm and leg didn't work. But I knew she was just saying that to please me.

She did begin to look to the left, to turn to the left, to see people on her left side, but she would sometimes sit and stare down at her hands with a strange questioning look in her eyes. And if I held up her left hand in my hand, she'd say she saw two hands and one was mine. But she couldn't tell me who the other one belonged to.

Betty never walked again. She could never even dress herself. She couldn't put on makeup, for if she tried, she always gave far more attention to the right half of her face than to the left. I can still see the results of one such effort; rouge only on the right cheek and lipstick that covered only two-thirds of her lips.

She would sit all day listening to music, opera mostly. Her vision was perfect, but she couldn't read, since she never saw the left half of the page. She sat and stared toward the right and listened to operas, no longer bothering to identify who was singing and never analyzing how well they were singing.

That was her condition when she left the hospital. She never got any better.

Some neurologist.

My mother and I talked about Betty's stroke only once about two years later. Betty finally developed pneumonia and died.

"There was nothing anyone could do for her," I said weakly.

"I know," my mother replied. "She saw the best neurologist, and even you couldn't help her."

Mothers are like that.

ADDENDUM

It's a long way from amphioxsis.

"Why," Barbara Phillips had once asked me, "does the left side of the brain control the right side of the body?"

I am always tempted to answer this rhetorical question, which I have used in teaching, by saying merely that God wanted it that way. It's the answer I believe, but I also believe in evolution and my job is to try to help students understand the brain and how it works, not the ways of God. Barbara deserved an explanation, not a biblical exegesis.

"Because," I explained, "the parietal eye of early amphibians had a lens."

I could tell that she had not grasped the full meaning of my answer, so I elucidated it.

On that long trip from amphioxsis to man, one stage was the amphibians. Many amphibians developed a single extra eye in the top of the head. This eye was above the parietal lobes, and is occasionally called the parietal eye, though because it served to transmit signals to the pineal area of the brain, it is more often called the pineal eye.

The pineal eye has a lens, and it's the lens that makes all the difference.

If an object, say some insect the amphibian would love to eat, moves from left to right, the image on the retina of the pineal eye also moves. If there were no lens, the image would move in the same direction. If there is a lens, however, the image moves the other way, to the left. The fly is now on the right. And the image is on the left side of the pineal retina and the left half of the brain. And the amphibian still wants to eat that fly.

To eat it, he must catch it; to catch it, he must see it. So as the fly moves farther to the right, he must turn his eye by lowering the right side. A muscle on the right side of the head must pull that lens down. But the sensation to trigger that movement is in the left brain. So the left brain has to send a nerve out to that muscle on the other side of the skull—from left to right. That phenomenon is called decussation, or crossing of nerve fibers, and it all started with the amphibians, the amphibians and God.

Sometimes a stroke on the left side is called a left-sided stroke because it involves a lesion on the left side of the brain. But because it causes a right hemiplegia, it's sometimes called a right-sided stroke. At times it can be very confusing.

The same Barbara Phillips once presented a complicated patient to me. She had spent much of the night chasing down the patient's history. She'd even called other hospitals to get the discharge summaries. The patient had at least five separate strokes. That's where the confusion set in. Barbara called one of the strokes left sided, and meant left side of the brain. Or did she mean left hemiplegia? And another was right sided. That meant right hemiplegia. Or did it?

I became lost.

"Barbara," I asked. "Tell me again. Where was the second stroke?"

"At Mount Sinai Hospital," she said without blinking an eye.

Author's Note

As far as I know, there are no good explanations of the function of the parietal lobes aimed at the educated general reader. At times, I'm convinced there are not even any good sources for neurologists. All in all, the best source probably is MacDonald Critchley's *The Parietal Lobes* (New York: Hafner, 1966).

2

Still Smiling

Youth emits smiles without any reason. It is one of its chiefest charms.
—Oscar Wilde, *The Picture of Dorian Gray*

Jane Porter had always been happy, even as a child. She was no longer a child when her parents brought her to my office, but a twenty-year-old woman, a second-year college student who had just failed all her courses and whose fiancé was threatening to call off their wedding, which was just two weeks off. She was no longer happy, but she was still smiling, nonetheless. According to her parents, she had always been bright. She'd started reading long before she entered kindergarten. She'd always been a good student. They could understand her indifference toward her fiancé, since he was not good enough or smart enough for her. But they could not understand her loss of interest in her schoolwork, in her friends, in them, or in life. All she did now was smile.

They had already taken her to see a series of doctors, none of whom had helped. They'd decided she was a schizophrenic and admitted her to the psychiatry service in the hospital. There, another doctor whom they had never met, had made another diagnosis: hebephrenia. Her parents were unwilling to give up. There had to be something that someone could do to help their daughter. If not a psychiatrist, perhaps a neurologist.

I shook my head, at least partially in disbelief. Hebephrenia is the rarest form of schizophrenia. It is so rare, in fact, that it had long ago become a standard joke among neurology residents. Traditionally, neurology residents had to learn psychiatry because it was included on the certifying examination for neurologists. To these residents, hebephrenia was the psychiatric equivalent of the gnu. In the same way that the natural habitat of the gnu was the crossword puzzle, the only place that hebephrenia occurred was on psychiatric board examinations—not in the real day-to-day world of medical practice.

One of the major features of hebephrenia is spontaneous, uncontrolled, inappropriate laughter; another is a bad prognosis. The patients never recover. A diagnosis of hebephrenia is like a sentence of life in prison but without the possibility of parole.

Did Jane Porter laugh a lot? Not according to her parents. She just smiled, and smiled for no reason.

I looked at her. Jane had not said a word yet. I nodded at her, and she smiled back at me. It was a peculiar smile—not friendly, not joyous, not happy, but there all the while. A smile that refused to fade. Closer to a sneer than a smile. A sardonic smile. In neurology, this condition is called by its Latin equivalent, *risus sardonicus.* Using Latin doesn't make neurologists any smarter, but it does serve to remind them that *risus sardonicus,* a fixed sardonic smile that does not go away, is a sign of a neurologic disease, not of a psychiatric disease per se.

But which neurologic disease did Jane have?

A *risus sardonicus* is seen in two different clinical settings. It can be one of the first signs of either tetanus or of strychnine poisoning. Both of these are acute, rapidly progressive disorders. Patients die of strychnine poisoning in minutes, hours at the most, and although tetanus can last for weeks, the patient is totally disabled within a week or two at the most.

"How long had she been smiling?" I asked.

"Months," I was told.

Strychnine poisoning and tetanus were out. That left only one possibility. She had a dystonia.

Dystonia is a word we use to characterize an entire group or class of abnormal involuntary movements to differentiate them from other forms of abnormal movements, such as tremor and chorea. Tremors are brief rhythmic motions that involve alternating movements of opposing muscles, which lead to a regular back-and-forth motion occurring many times per second. Chorea consists of random, nonrepetitive, nonrhythmic, brief muscle jerks that form no pattern. Dystonias (dystonic movements), in contrast, are movements that cause an abnormal posture, which is then maintained for seconds or longer. If the neck or limbs are involved, there is invariably a rotational or torsion component in the resulting posture. A dystonia of the neck, for example, causes the head and neck to turn to one side. This condition is called torticollis (torsion or turning of the neck). Because they have no axis on which to turn, and thus cannot cause torsion, the muscles of the face merely present abnormal fixed postures in dystonia.

Risus sardonicus is a dystonia, an abnormal movement resulting in a fixed posture that lasts for seconds or more. In this case, far more: Jane was still smiling at me.

"Are you happy?" I asked.

"Noth," she slurred at me.

"Do you like smiling?"

She shook her head. It started as a simple shake, but suddenly she lost control, and her head pulled back violently. As that happened, her smile became more forceful. It was no longer a sneer, but now more like a silent, hysterical laugh. A grotesque of a real laugh. This new posture lasted almost thirty seconds, and then her head returned to its normal position. "Noth," she answered, as her smile began to fade back toward her usual sneer.

I had now identified one physical symptom (her smile), and instead of merely using a Latin descriptive phrase, I had classified it as a type of abnormal movement labeled under another latinized rubric. That might not seem like much progress, but it is.

One of the great triumphs of late nineteenth- and early twentieth-century neurology was the clear differentiation of these separate classes of abnormal movements. It was a major advance because the two classes represent distinct diseases with specific pathologies involving different parts of the brain. Most important, each of these separate diseases has a different cause and today, of course, its own form of treatment. This process was so important and recognized as such by contemporaries that the names of the clinicians who first clearly delineated the disorders became attached to "their" respective diseases.

It was James Parkinson who described the rhythmic rest tremor of what he called *paralysis agitans,* or the shaking palsy. We call it Parkinson's disease. George Huntington described hereditary chorea with dementia and insanity. We call it Huntington's chorea or Huntington's disease. Samuel A. K. Wilson described dystonia with liver disease, which he called "progressive lenticular degeneration," and we call Wilson's disease. The one exception is Hermann Oppenheim. He first described dystonia as part of a disease he called dystonia musculorum deformans. We still call it dystonia musculorum deformans (DMD for short), although Oppenheim's disease would be easier to say.

So I now knew the class of disorders Jane had, but which particular form of dystonia afflicted her? More than one disease can cause dystonic movements. Did she have DMD? Or Wilson's disease? Or something else? Wilson's disease involves both the brain and the liver. Was her liver normal?

"Did the doctors find anything else?" I asked.

"No," her mother sighed weakly.

"Are you certain?" I interrupted.

"Nothing," she said. "The brain wave test was normal and the skull X rays. Nothing."

"How about the liver tests?"

"They said that didn't matter. Her liver was fine."

"What didn't matter?" I persisted.

"The liver tests. Her liver's okay."

"Were the tests normal?" I demanded.

"They weren't high enough to cause her problem."

That had not been the question. "Were they normal?" I repeated.

"No. They weren't." With that she handed me the list of lab tests.

I looked them over.

Jane had abnormal liver function. Her abnormalities were mild—that was true—and certainly not bad enough to suggest that liver failure was causing her changed behavior. But her tests were definitely abnormal, and the abnormalities were of the type that are found in cirrhosis of the liver. The title of Wilson's original paper leapt to mind: "Progressive Lenticular Degeneration: A Familiar Nervous Disease Associated with Cirrhosis of the Liver."

Wilson's disease: A curable disease if diagnosed correctly and early enough.

I took Jane into the examining room and began by asking her to tell me her story in her own words. It was not a pleasant one and telling it was not an easy task. Her speech was slurred and slow, and if she tried to speak loudly, her words became forced and her sentences choppy, until it was almost impossible for her to understand her own words.

Her problems were symptoms of her disease, I said, trying to reassure her.

"Soth. I amth crathy."

"No. No. Not at all. I guarantee that. You have a neurologic disease."

"I'm noth justh crathy?"

"No. You are not crazy at all."

She looked up at me and began to cry and as she did so, her head flew back, and that same hideous broad grin I had seen before once again contorted her face. Her eyes sprang fully open, and her tongue burst out of her mouth as if she were about to vomit.

In about a minute she was back to her usual *risus sardonicus*.

She'd been valedictorian of her class in high school. She'd decided to stay at home to go to college. Her boyfriend was there, working as a car mechanic. He was smart but he didn't like school. During her first year, she received all As, and her parents agreed to let her get married as long as she promised to finish college. The couple didn't need her parents' consent, for Jane was old enough, but their approval was important to her. The wedding was set for the coming June, after she finished her second year of college.

She never completed it. It seemed so much harder than her freshman year had been, right from the beginning—especially French. And she'd always been so good at languages. She had planned to major in Romance languages: French, Spanish, and Italian. It was French that she loved the most, that had always been easy for her. That all changed. She started to have trouble with enunciation and as the first semester went on, she went from bad to worse. Her French pronunciation had always been perfect. She'd often tutored the other students in the language lab.

Her parents blamed Scott. Scott was putting pressure on her. He didn't want to wait any longer. After all, they were engaged.

She agreed. She didn't want to wait, either. So they stopped waiting. That pressure was gone. It didn't help.

Her pronunciation grew worse, until even her English deteriorated. She flunked French and Italian.

Her parents couldn't understand what was happening to her, and neither could she.

The second semester started. By now, everything was harder—impossible, in fact. She flunked all her midterm exams.

She lost interest in everything, and everyone. She stopped calling her friends, and they stopped calling her. She didn't want to make love anymore, and didn't even want to see Scott.

That was when she began to be convinced that she was losing her mind—that she was going crazy—and the doctors confirmed her worst fears.

Schizophrenia.

Hebephrenia.

She wasn't sure what either of those terms really meant, except that she was crazy and they could not help her.

Once again, in the course of her story, she began to cry. Not tears of happiness this time, but tears of fright. Once again, her head reared back, and that grotesque smile forced itself upon her. With it came a sudden, forced, deep breath and a loud gasp that echoed through the small examining room, like the laugh of an uncontrolled hebephrenic.

"You are not schizophrenic," I began. "Nor hebephrenic. You have dystonia."

That was another term she did not understand. I explained it to her and explained how dystonia movements are brought on by muscle activity, especially newly learned or difficult actions. Dystonia of the muscles of speech is brought on by speech. The louder you speak, the worse the dystonia. The softer, the better.

She heard what I said, and it made sense to her.

I told her to count from one to ten loudly.

"Onth. Tooth!" This came out as a short word, more a grunt than a word.

She stopped with a smile, a gasp.

"Tree. Fort." More a bark than a word.

I stopped her. "Now," I said. "Whisper from one to ten." I put my ear in front of her lips.

"One, two, three, four," she began. No stops. No grunts. No barks. No slurs.

At twenty, I stopped her.

"Dystonia," I said.

"Dystonia," she whispered back to me. "Can you cure me?" she asked in her newfound whisper.

"I must check one thing," I replied.

I looked at her eyes, not with my ophthalmoscope but with my own naked eyes.

I could cure her.

"Yes," I said. "You have Wilson's disease, and that we can treat."

I brought her back into my office and explained what I now knew to both her and her parents.

Wilson's disease is very rare. When I saw Jane in 1975, I had already been specializing in movement disorder for six or seven years. I had seen hundreds of patients with Parkinson's disease and scores with Huntington's disease. She was the first person I had encountered with Wilson's disease.

Wilson's disease, I explained to them, is a hereditary disease.

But, the parents protested, no one else in the family had any neurologic problems.

Were they sure?

They were sure.

I explained how that could be true. Jane had only one sibling, a younger brother. The gene for Wilson's disease is recessive. To get Wilson's disease, you have to inherit its gene from both your parents—one from each parent. This means that each parent has to be a carrier. The gene occurs in about one out of every hundred individuals so it is unlikely that anyone else in either family who might have been carrying one abnormal gene would have married someone else with the gene. As a result, most patients do not have a history of relatives with similar problems.

Wilson's disease is a disorder in the way the body handles copper. Normally, copper is absorbed from the intestine. It is loosely bound in the blood with various proteins, especially albumin. This loosely bound copper then circulates throughout the body, with most of it eventually taken up by the liver. Every tissue needs copper, for it is a necessary constituent of numerous enzymes. The copper that is taken up by the liver is incorporated in a protein called ceruloplasmin. Cerulo means blue and is derived from the bluish color that copper gives to this protein. No one knows what ceruloplasmin does.

In Wilson's disease, the process goes haywire. More copper is absorbed through the gut than is normally needed. The liver doesn't take up this excess, and, as a result, a lot more loosely bound copper is distributed to the other tissues. When the levels of copper in the tissues become too high, the organs begin to degenerate. Two parts of the body are particularly susceptible to this form of copper poisoning: the brain and the liver. In the brain, this causes dystonia, loss of intellectual functions, and personality changes. In the liver, it causes cirrhosis.

Was I sure Jane had Wilson's disease?

Yes, for I could see the copper. It was not just in her liver and her brain, but had spread throughout her system. One place its presence was visible was her eyes, her irises. In Wilson's disease, the copper is deposited as a greenish-colored ring around the outer edge of the cornea. These rings are called Kayser-Fleischer rings after the two neurologists who first detected them.

That didn't seem to be quite enough for Jane's parents. Could I prove that their daughter had Wilson's disease? They'd already been through schizophrenia and hebephrenia.

There were, fortunately, methods of confirming the diagnosis. In Wilson's disease, the ceruloplasmin level is low. Measuring that level is the first step. A low ceruloplasmin proves that the liver is not taking up copper and making ceruloplasmin. The next step is the proof. Wilson's disease is, in a sense, merely copper poisoning. The final proof is the detection of abnormally high levels of copper in the tissues. Seeing the Kayser-Fleischer rings is one such test. The next, one that provides those chemical numbers on which patients and doctors prefer to rely, even though they are neither more accurate nor more reliable than Kayser-Fleischer rings, involves performing a liver biopsy and measuring the actual amount of copper present in the organ. If the level of copper is elevated, it confirms the diagnosis of Wilson's disease.

That, Jane's family understood.

Next we'd do a CAT scan, which would give us an idea of degree of permanent brain injury, if any. Then we would start treatment.

Jane was admitted to the hospital two days later. We evaluated her blood ceruloplasmin. It was too low to be detectable.

We performed a liver biopsy. The copper level in the liver was abnormally high—six times the upper limit of normal. Everyone was convinced; Jane had Wilson's disease.

What could be done for her? A lot. Her CAT scan revealed little evidence of permanent injury. Her prognosis was excellent.

The first successful treatment of Wilson's disease was a chemical called BAL, or British Anti-Lewisite. Lewisite was a poison that contained arsenic; BAL was developed to remove arsenic from the tissues of victims of Lewisite poisoning. BAL or dimercaprol has two sulphydryl groups. These are chemical groups that contain a sulfur and a hydrogen atom. The sulfur atom has a high affinity for many metallic ions. It pulls these ions out of the tissues into which they have become bound, and the metal-containing BAL molecule is excreted out of the body in the urine. The drug works the same way in Wilson's disease, except now the BAL removes copper instead of arsenic.

BAL was the first medication that gave us the potential of curing what had been considered to be an incurable disease. Because it caused too many side effects, however, it was eventually replaced by penicillamine, another simple chemical that is able to draw copper out of the body.

I started Jane on penicillamine. Our problems were not over, I told her parents. We had to make sure that Jane's brother didn't have the same disease.

What were his odds? One out of four. I drew it out for them as we do in text books: A lower-case w represents the normal gene. An upper-case W represents the abnormal gene for Wilson's disease. Jane had two genes for Wilson's disease: WW.

Each parent had one gene: wW.

Jane's heritage would be represented this way:

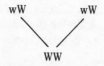

Since the lining up of genes in the genetic process is random, each time one of her father's sperm and one of her mother's eggs met, there were four possible genetic combinations:

w (maternal)—w (paternal)

w (maternal)—W (paternal)

W (maternal)—w (paternal)

W (maternal)—W (paternal)

In other words, the chances were as follows:

ww	normal	25 percent
wW or Ww	a potential carrier	50 percent
WW	Wilson's disease	25 percent

One out of four.

The following week, I saw Jane's brother. He had no neurologic symptoms, no Kayser-Fleischer rings, and his ceruloplasmin was normal. He did not have Wilson's disease. He might still be a carrier, but unless he married another carrier, it would make no difference. And the odds were 200 to 1 against his doing so.

Jane improved rapidly. In six months, she was back in school and doing well. In a year she was back tutoring in French. She eventually received a Ph.D. in romance languages and is a tenured associate professor of French at one of the Big Ten universities. She never did marry Scott who was frightened of the concept of a hereditary disease. In 1978, Jane married a fellow graduate student, and now has two children. Both the children are carriers; they had to be. All Jane had to give them genetically were Ws. But they both have normal levels of ceruloplasmin. The odds are 200 to 1 that being carriers will make no difference in their lives nor the lives of their children. Jane Porter still has Wilson's disease. She always will. She remains on treatment and is free of any symptoms.

When Jane was in the hospital, she was seen by all the residents, none of whom had ever come across a patient with Wilson's disease. After they had all seen her, I held a teaching conference on Wilson's disease. By that time, they had all read up on Wilson's disease and thought they knew all the answers.

"What," I asked my senior resident, "did Wilson see in the eyes of his patients?"

"Kayser-Fleischer rings," she replied.

"Nothing," I corrected her. "If he'd seen them, we'd call them Wilson's rings. But he didn't see them."

"Why not?" she asked.

"He never looked."

I could not fault Wilson for not looking. There was no reason for him to suspect that he would see anything abnormal on the outer edge of the iris. It is not a symptom that occurs in other diseases.

But today there is no excuse for oversight.

Jane's psychiatrists should have looked at her irises or asked someone else to look. In fact, they described her eyes as WNL. In the shorthand of medical recordkeeping, WNL is one of the most widely used acronyms. It is supposed to mean "within normal limits." Unfortunately, it often means "We never looked."

My resident now asked me a question. Did I know why Jane deteriorated so much more quickly after she and Scott had started making love?

I had no answer. I had not even given that problem much thought.

But the resident had an answer. "Her form of contraception."

I looked at her skeptically.

"She used an IUD," I was told.

"So what?"

"She used a copper-7. And copper is absorbed from a copper-7. More copper made her disease worse."

She was right. I'd never asked Jane about contraception. In my generation, we were taught not to ask such questions except as a last resort, if then. Fortunately, medicine has changed.

Author's Note

Hermann Oppenheim (1858-1919) was the leader of German neurology during the latter part of the nineteenth century and the early part of the twentieth. His textbook *Lehrbuch der Nervenkrankheiten* was a significant landmark in the development of neurology. Oppenheim was also the first German-born neurologist to feel the effects of the official government anti-Semitism in Germany. Born in Warburg, Westphalia, he studied medicine at three leading German universities: Göttingen, Berlin, and Bonn. After graduation, he became an assistant first at a psychiatric clinic at the Charité, Berlin's largest hospital and part of the University of Berlin. There he studied with Carl Westphal (1833-90), who wrote the first description of the knee jerk in 1875. Beginning as Westphal's assistant, Oppenheim soon became his associate and actually took charge of the department during

Westphal's long terminal illness. Following Westphal's death, Oppenheim was not given Westphal's position of professor at the Charité; instead, he was forced through anti-Semitism to leave that august institution and open his own private clinic. On Westphal's death, the medical faculty of the University of Berlin unanimously nominated Oppenheim to succeed Westphal as Professor Extraordinarius, a nomination that the Prussian secretary of education adamantly refused to confirm.

Despite such difficulties, Oppenheim was able to rise to a position of leadership among German neurologists. He never held an official teaching post, never again held a post in any state institution, and was deprived of the opportunity to teach within the established system. Instead of following the usual academic pathway, Oppenheim carved out his scientific career independently. His private clinic soon became an international referral center for clinical neurology, and his prolific mind and pen produced numerous important publications.

3

Newton's Madness

Madness in great ones must not unwatched go.
— Shakespeare, *Hamlet*

We are all born mad. Some remain so.
— Samuel Beckett, *Waiting for Godot*

Sir Isaac Newton is one of the few scientists in the history of Western civilization whose reputation is universal and whose name is synonymous with genius. Newton, Aristotle, Einstein—I doubt if there are many others. Newton lived from 1642 to 1727. Today he is considered to have been a natural philosopher. He was actually a physicist and mathematician and, with the possible exception of Albert Einstein, he may well have been the most original and influential theorist in the history of science. His list of accomplishments is impressive:

1. The coinvention of calculus. Working independently, Newton and Gottfried Wilhelm Leibniz both "invented," or discovered, calculus.
2. The discovery of the three laws of mechanics (Newton's laws) which transformed the entire field of physics.
3. The formulation of the law of gravity.
4. The discovery of the composition of white light.
5. The formulation of a theory of planetary motion.

The list does not end there, but my purpose here is not to investigate the mind of Sir Isaac Newton and the influence of that mind on Western civilization. Rather, it is to explore the nature and cause of Newton's madness and its effect on Newton the man and Newton the scientist. For Newton became mad. Not permanently deranged, but twice during his life, he suffered periods of prolonged abnormal behavior, bordering on psychosis. His madness was of his own doing, and it was a malady that did not leave him unscathed.

The first episode of his madness lasted through most of 1677 and 1678, while the second began in 1693. The former is not as well documented in contemporary records, for it came at a time in his career when he was not yet a public figure. Newton's symptoms of "madness" began at about the time of his first scientific publication concerning his theory of the composition of white light. Newton himself considered this work to be "the oddest if not the most considerable detection which has hitherto been made in operations of Nature." His paper was not immediately accepted by the entire scientific community and Newton's reactions to the criticisms of this work were not the logical reactions of a finely tuned genius. Newton scholar Richard S. Westfall studied these responses and suggested that Newton's behavior showed definite signs of abnormality. Westfall was particularly struck by Newton's correspondence with a critic named John Lucas:

> The correspondence dragged on until 1678, when a final shriek of rage from Newton, apparently accompanied by a complete nervous breakdown, was followed by silence. The death of his mother the following year completed his isolation. For six years he withdrew from intellectual commerce, except when others initiated a correspondence, which he always broke off as soon as possible.

It was not until 1684 that Newton once again began to seek the company of others and to interact with fellow scientists.

Although most studies of Newton's life have passed over this first instance of altered behavior, it is generally acknowledged in both the historical and scientific communities that in the years 1692 and 1693, Newton underwent a period of severe emotional and mental disturbance. This entire episode has always had about it something of an air of mystery. The first biography of Newton, published in London and Paris in 1728, the year after Newton's death, was written by a Frenchman named Bernard Le Bovier de Fontenelle, who was the permanent secretary of the Academie Royale des Sciences. Le Bovier de Fontenelle based his work largely on information and material given to him by John Conduitt. Conduitt was married to Newton's niece and had spent many years and much energy collecting materials for a projected biography of Newton that he intended to write but that he never undertook. Whatever he gave to Fontenelle contained no reference to any mental disorder suffered by Newton. Either Conduitt was ignorant of this episode or he knew of it but decided to suppress it—the latter being far more likely. Fontenelle's biography was widely read and, since it was based on contemporary source material, it became the primary foundation of virtually all subsequent studies of Newton's life. For the next hundred years, no biographies even hinted at the possibility of a mental illness.

In 1820, this viewpoint began to change. In that year, the French astronomer Jean Baptiste Biot wrote a sketch of Newton for the *Biographie Universelle,* in which he stated that in 1693, Newton suffered what Biot termed a "derangement of the intellect," during which his "reason" was abnormal.

Much of the proof that this "derangement of the intellect" actually took place became readily available only in 1961 when Volume 3 of Newton's correspondence, covering the years 1688 through 1694, was finally published. Most accounts of Newton's illness have dated its onset to late 1693. However, a careful study of his correspondence reveals definite signs of emotional stress beginning at least eighteen months earlier. On January 26, 1692, Newton, who was then living in Cambridge, complained to John Locke that his old and hitherto completely loyal friend, Charles Montague, had been false to him, and that he, Newton, was "done with him." The same distrust is revealed in other letters written at the same time.

Whether the conflicts that Newton experienced in his relationship with Montague, Locke, and others were real or imaginary, we have no way of proving, but since numerous relationships were similarly affected at the same time, the odds are that the problem originated in Newton's mind or behavior. For the next eighteen months, the letters reveal nothing out of the ordinary.

Beginning on May 30, 1693, there is a period of three and a half months of silence, during which we have no record of any letter either received or written by Newton. The silence was finally interrupted by correspondence in which he exhibited the peculiar sensitivity that had been present during the early months of the previous years, but in a far more intensified form. Newton sent the following strange letter to the famous diarist Samuel Pepys on September 13, 1693:

Sir,

Some time after Mr. Millington had delivered your message, he pressed me to see you the next time I went to London. I was averse; but upon his pressing consented, before I considered what I did, for I am extremely trou-

bled at the embroilment I am in, and have neither ate nor slept well this
twelve month, nor have my former consistency of mind. I never designed to
get anything by your interest, nor by King James's favour, but am now
sensible that I must withdraw from your acquaintance, and see neither you
nor the rest of my friends any more, if I may but leave them quietly. I beg
your pardon for saying I would see you again, and rest your most humble
and most obedient servant,

Is. Newton

The same year, Newton wrote to Locke: "being of the opinion that you
endeavoured to embroil me with women and by other means I was so much
affected with it as that when one told me that you were sickly and would
not live I answered twere better you were dead. I desire you to forgive me
this uncharitableness." Both Pepys and Locke recognized that Newton's
mind was deranged, and in other letters it is clear that his memory was
also impaired.

These symptoms are reminiscent of those of his first episode of madness,
which also resulted in Newton's withdrawing from society: suspiciousness
of others, accusations, and withdrawal.

What, in fact, caused these two breakdowns?

Did Newton have a recurring psychosis—such as manic depressive affec-
tive disorder—with two separate and distinct psychotic breaks? Or were
there specific factors in his life that precipitated each of these periods of
psychological maladjustment?

Most of Newton's twentieth-century biographers have focused on the
latter and have suggested a staggering number of hypotheses to explain the
precipitation of one or the other of these episodes:

1. The shock of his mother's death. This hypothesis is all very Freud-
   ian. Unfortunately, Mrs. Newton died in 1679, too late to account
   for the first episode and too early for the second.
2. A fire that destroyed some important papers.
3. Failure to obtain a desired administrative post in London.
4. Exhaustion following the writing of his *Principia*.
5. Religious fervor.
6. Local problems with the university at Cambridge.

The list goes on and on. I will attempt neither to document them all
nor to refute them one by one. Instead, I will invoke what I sometimes
call "Baker's law." Baker's law is a law that I have propounded out of
one of A. B. Baker's irrascible bedside pronouncements. A. B. Baker, one

of the leading figures of American neurology in the middle third of this century, was primarily responsible for the founding of the American Academy of Neurology, which has, in fewer than forty years, become the leading force in American and world neurology, and one of the founders of *Neurology,* the first American medical journal dedicated solely to the field. He was also the chairman of neurology at the University of Minnesota, where I began my formal training in neurology.

Abe Baker was a clinician who shot from the hip. During a typical teaching session, one of my fellow first-year residents was presenting a patient who had a confusional psychosis. After telling Abe about the entire medical history of this patient and the results of the physical examination, this poor, unsuspecting resident then began to recount the patient's psychiatric history. Abe would have none of it. He exploded. A psychiatric history is a waste of time, he said. No neurologist should ever take one. Everybody has psychiatric problems. The whole world is crazy, so are all its inhabitants. The question is not if a patient has a psychiatric problem. The question is whether the patient has a neurologic problem that can account for his or her behavior. That is a neurologic question and has to be evaluated on neurologic grounds, not on psychiatric ones. A psychiatric history is irrelevant.

Thus, Baker's law: The entire neurologic issue is whether the patient has a neurologic disease or not. All else is mere commentary.

Did Newton have a neurologic problem that could account for his psychosis. If he did, his mother's death is irrelevant. If not, then his mother's death is a subject for psychiatrists to debate.

What evidence is there that Newton could have had a neurologic disorder? From his correspondence, a list of his signs and symptoms, both neurologic and psychiatric, can easily be compiled. They include

1. Severe insomnia
2. Extreme sensitivity in personal relations
3. Loss of appetite
4. Delusions of persecution
5. Memory difficulties
6. Some overall decrease in mental acuity

This is certainly the type of behavioral manifestation that can be seen in a variety of diffuse processes that cause mild (neurologically speaking) alteration in the function of both hemispheres of the brain. It is a neurologic rule of thumb that generalized behavioral symptoms such as these are usually related to diffuse or generalized dysfunction of the entire brain, that is, both halves, rather than just disease in a single location. Diseases that affect a single site in the brain, in contrast, cause symptoms that are related specifically to the normal function carried out by that location: weakness, speech difficulty, and loss of vision.

Because behaviors like memory, concentration, intellect, and judgment are not localized in one spot, they are more likely to become deranged in mild diffuse diseases that insult the brain generally without singling out any one specific locus.

A neurologic cause is, therefore, plausible as an explanation for Newton's odd behavior. But what cause? In recent years, two separate scientific reports have suggested that Newton's madness was caused by chronic mercury poisoning and that the poisoning was self-induced, a product of Newton's interest in alchemy.

Two English scientists named Spargo and Pounds conducted a careful examination of the records of Newton's chemical experiments. Newton had shown an interest in alchemy and chemistry and had even purchased a variety of apparatuses and chemicals as early as 1669. His last dated chemical experiments were carried out in February 1696, not long before he left Cambridge and moved to London. During his many years in Cambridge, Newton carried out several hundred chemical experiments, of which only a small number were specifically dated. However, from those that are dated, it is clear that Newton ran many of his experiments shortly before the first signs of each of his episodes of "madness." Newton made use of a wide variety of materials in his chemical research, including nonmetallic materials, such as sulfur, "sal armoniak" (ammonium chloride), and sulfuric and nitric acids, and metals, such as antimony, mercury, iron, tin, bismuth, lead, "arsnick," and copper, as well as many of their ores. Metals tended to play a prominent role in virtually all Newton's experiments, and mercury in particular was a major component in many of his studies.

In many of his experiments, Newton heated metals, their ores, or their salts to convert them into a volatile form. He would often heat these substances in open vessels, breathing in the fumes and tasting the formed products. Some of these experiments were simple and took little time, while others were complex and extended over many hours or, in a few cases, even days. While conducting research, Newton regularly slept in his laboratory by the same fire, which did not go out for weeks on end. Since most of the volatized metal fumes would have settled back into the fire only to be volatilized again, this clearly exposed him to an additional risk of metallic poisoning.

Newton conducted a number of alchemical experiments in December

1692 and January 1693, in which he used antimony, antimony ore, and a "mercurial water of lead," which was probably a lead amalgam. In these experiments a saltlike substance appeared in the neck of the retort. After reporting the taste of this substance under two conditions, he then continued: "I held it to ye side of ye flame of candle and it did not take flame as [sulphur] would do but yet fumed away and ye fumes made the side of ye flame look blue."

Information about Newton's working habits in chemistry is also found in the recollections of his assistant, Humphrey Newton:

> He very rarely went to bed till two or three of the clock, sometimes not until five or six, lying about four or five hours, especially at spring or the fall of the leaf, at which time he would employ about six weeks in his laboratory, the fire scarcely going out either night or day, he sitting up, one night as I did another, till he had finished his chemical experiments, in the performance of which he was the most accurate, strict, exact. What his aim might be I was not able to penetrate into, but his pains, his diligence at those set times made me think he aimed at something beyond the reach of human art or industry.

> About six weeks at spring, and six in the fall, the fire in the elaboratory scarcely went out, which was well furnished with chemical materials as bodies, receivers, heads, crucibles, etc., which was [sic] made very little use of, the crucibles excepted, in which he fused his metals: he would sometimes, tho' seldom, look into an old mouldy book which lay in his elaboratory, I think it was titled Agricola de metallis, the transmuting of metals being his chief design.

Tasting mercury compounds and breathing the fumes of its various salts is highly hazardous. Metallic fumes are one of the most efficient ways of introducing an excessive amount of a metal into the body, since they enter the lungs and are quickly absorbed. It was at this point that Newton began to suffer from poor digestion and insomnia. It is even possible that Newton himself identified the cause of his symptoms as exposure to the quicksilver (mercury) vapors. After all, its effects had been known to alchemical writers for centuries before Newton, and Newton was quite familiar with their writings. In the following passage, Newton hints at the correct diagnosis of his malady:

> The last winter by sleeping too often by my fire I got into an ill habit of sleeping and a distemper which this summer has been epidemical put me further out of order, so that when I wrote to you I had not slept an hour a night for a fortnight together and for five nights together not a wink. I

remember I wrote to you but what I said of your book I remember not. If you please to send me a transcript of that passage I will give you an account of it if I can.

Obviously, Newton was exposed to metallic mercury in 1692–93. Was that also the case in 1676? The answer is yes. The experiments he performed in connection with his study of "optiks" often involved significant exposure to mercury vapors, and during the period 1676–79 he also began a period of intense study of alchemy.

The exposure is proved. Newton was at risk for mercury poisoning. But does mercury poisoning cause madness?

In his 1964 textbook on mercury poisoning, *The Toxicity of Mercury and Its Compounds* (Amsterdam: Elsevier), Peter Bidstrup supplied the following description of chronic mercury poisoning: "Nervous irritability, tendency to blush easily, and a history—often best obtained from friends or members of the family—of change of temperament, a tendency to avoid meeting friends and unexplained outbursts of temper."

This description certainly reminds us of Newton. Of course, the initial symptoms of mercury poisoning differ from patient to patient. In 1893, the great English neurologist William R. Gowers investigated the syndrome of chronic mercury poisoning and pointed out that it often begins with irritability and difficulty with concentration, followed by insomnia and finally by hallucinations and maniacal excitement. There is frequently a compelling, overwhelming timidness; a shyness of strangers; an embarrassment about the illness; discouragement and apathy about all aspects of life (but not despair); a loss of self-confidence; a loss of joie de vivre progressing to depression; and finally, a loss of memory.

The key to suspecting that a patient undergoing such a personality change has a neurologic disorder is the appearance of neurologic signs and symptoms. In mercury poisoning, the most common of these is a tremor.

And Newton had a tremor: His handwriting in 1692–93 became tremulous, while before and afterward, it was firm and precise.

We are now two-thirds of the way to diagnosis.

1. Newton had sufficient exposure.
2. Newton had a clinical picture that is consistent with mercury poisoning, including neurologic findings.

But what good is a hypothesis unless it can be tested? Not much. It is the last step that is critical in reaching a diagnosis. Is there any way to prove that Newton actually had a toxic amount of mercury in his body?

Spargo and Pounds did just that. Today, we often diagnose mercury poisoning by measuring the amount of mercury present in the urine, the blood, or the hair. Obviously, the first two cannot be evaluated for Newton, but Spargo and Pounds were able to locate several locks of his hair. In them they found clear evidence of excessive amounts of mercury.

Abe was right: Baker's law at work. The diagnosis could have been made on neurologic grounds, without the need of taking a psychiatric history.

What happened to Newton following his second episode of madness?

In 1696, Newton moved to London and became master of the mint, leaving Cambridge—and alchemy—behind him. During his London years, he enjoyed both power and worldly success. His position at the mint assured a comfortable social and economic status, and he was an active and able administrator. After the death of Robert Hooke, the great microscopist, in 1703, Newton was elected president of the Royal Society and was annually reelected to this post until his death. In 1704, he published his second major work, the *Opticks,* based entirely on work completed decades before. In 1705, he was knighted by Queen Anne who, according to Conduitt, believed that it was her good fortune to have lived at the same time as, and to have known, so great a man. In London, "he reigned as the most famous man of his age, of Europe, and—as his powers gradually waned and his affability increased—perhaps of all time, so it seemed to his contemporaries" (Conduitt). In the more than 30 years that he lived in London, after leaving Cambridge, his illness (insomnia, loss of appetite, loss of memory, melancholia, delusions of persecution, and possibly trembling of the hands, as seen in his writing) appears to have been for the most part forgotten. But he never recovered his former level of function, spoke little in company, and was rather languid in his look and manner.

Although his creative years had passed, Newton continued to exercise a profound influence on the development of science. In effect, the Royal Society was his instrument, and he played it to his personal advantage. His tenure as president has been described as tyrannical and autocratic, and his control over the lives and careers of younger disciples was all but absolute. Newton could not abide contradiction or controversy and marshaled all the forces at his command in his various disputes. In his battle with Leibniz over who had priority in the discovery of calculus, Newton enlisted younger men to fight his war of words, while behind the lines he secretly directed charge and countercharge. In the end, the actions of the society were little more than extensions of Newton's will, and until his death he dominated all science without rival.

Looking over his entire career, it seems likely that his two episodes of mercury poisoning left their scars. His recovery was probably not complete, and Newton was left less overwhelmingly brilliant than he had once been, and tainted by a paranoid, hypersensitive streak.

This cannot be proved, nor can it be disproved.

But it fits the facts.

To me the most impressive part of this tale is not the fact that Newton developed mercury poisoning; after all, his exposure to mercury was significant. Nor is it the fact that scientific sleuthing done two hundred years after Newton's death has been able to find evidence that he did indeed suffer from mental aberrations due to his mercury exposure. It is the fact that despite these episodes of prolonged toxicity to his brain, he still retained sufficient intellectual capacity to remain the greatest intellect of his age.

Author's Note

The fact that mercury poisoning causes madness has long been suspected, and by the late nineteenth century it was part of general medical knowledge. In those times mercury was used in the felt-hat industry as a "carrot" or stiffening agent, and the most characteristic symptom of its workers was a tremor called "Hatters" shakes in the United Kingdom and Danbury Shakes in the United States. Since this condition was often accompanied by mental aberrations, Lewis Carroll based his character the Mad Hatter in *Alice in Wonderland* on a hatter whose madness was caused by mercury poisoning.

The two scientific articles that identified mercury poisoning as the cause of Newton's madness are these:

1. I. W. Johnson and M. L. Wolbarsht, "Mercury Poisoning: A Probable Cause of Isaac Newton's Physical and Mental Ills." *Notes Records of the Royal Society of London* 34 (1979): 1–9.

2. P. E. Spargo and C. A. Pounds, "Newton's 'Derangement of the Intellect': A New Light on an Old Problem." *Notes Records of the Royal Society of London* 34 (1979): 11–32.

The scientific analysis given here is based primarily on their discoveries. (The quotations from Newton's correspondence come from these secondary sources.) The best discussion of Newton's first mental crisis was presented by Robert F. Westfall *(Isis* 57 [1966]: 299–307).

A. B. Baker died in 1988. An obituary summarizing his contributions to neurology was published in *Neurology* (38 [1988]: 456). It makes no mention of Baker's law.

4

A Trip to Paradise

All you, healthy people, do not even suspect what happiness is, that happiness which we epileptics experience during the second before the attack. In his Koran Mohammed assures us that he saw paradise and was inside. All clever fools are convinced that he is simply a liar and a fraud. Oh no! He is not lying! He really was in paradise during an attack of epilepsy from which he suffered as I do. I don't know whether this bliss lasts seconds, hours or months, yet take my word for it, I would not exchange it for all the joys which life can give.

—Fyodor Mikailovich Dostoyevski

I was not the first neurologist whom Claudia Magee had consulted. Nor would I be the last. She let me know that fact as soon as she sat down in my office. As far as I could tell, her visits to numerous doctors were due to factors that were beyond her control. Or to be more precise, one factor—her husband Ned, who was in the middle of his journey up the corporate ladder. Claudia and Ned had started in Rochester, New York, with stops in Atlanta, Cleveland, Minneapolis, and several other towns before they had reached Chicago and she had come to me, having gotten my name from a former resident of mine who had been her neurologist during her short stay in a suburb just outside St. Louis.

Without my asking, she supplied a number of significant facts. She was thirty-three years old. I would have guessed her to be closer to forty. She was thin, and although she dressed quite fashionably, her clothes could not disguise the rather haggard tone in her appearance. She had four children ranging in age from six to two, which may have explained her haggard look. She refused to have any help in the house: she hated strangers, and when you moved as often as she did, the help were always strangers.

So her home situation did account for her looks. But did it explain her anger, which seemed to envelop her entire life, and would obviously soon extend to me—this strange new neurologist whom she had to consult as she continued her life as an upwardly mobile corporate gypsy? I suddenly recalled the man who taught me neuroanatomy. He had been at Minnesota for twenty years before he came to Chicago. When he told his wife they were moving, she told him that if they were going to move that frequently, they might as well just buy a trailer.

Claudia was, she continued, in perfect health.

And what was the problem that brought her to see so many neurologists? I inquired. The fact that she considered herself to be in perfect health eliminated any number of diagnostic possibilities. People with multiple sclerosis do not consider themselves to be in good health, nor do those with most other neurologic diseases. There were really only two possibilities: seizures and headaches. Please God, I said to myself, let it be migraine headaches. I could then send her off to another ex-resident of mine who specialized in that area and whose office was in the same building as mine. He could deal with her anger and its relationship to her headaches. That wasn't for me.

"I have complex partial seizures," she announced.

I knew I was in trouble. She had seen enough neurologists to know our lingo. But knowing the right phrases doesn't guarantee real understanding—far from it. However, it's often impossible to tell that to an angry patient, especially if the patient has already seen a half dozen other neurologists and already knows exactly what she has.

"What's a complex partial seizure?" I asked.

Her eyes flew open, and the creases on her forehead deepened, as did her crow's feet. "Perhaps I'm in the wrong place."

"No, Mrs. Magee. You're in the right place. I do know the answer. But do you?"

"Of course I do. It's the kind of seizure I have."

That was not an acceptable answer. I could either let it drop there and leave her in control or do it my way. I had no choice. The treatment of any chronic disease—and complex partial seizures that have required the care of a series of neurologists fit into that category—requires a working physician/patient relationship. The easiest way to start forging that relationship would have been for me to back away. But I happen to believe that a good physician/patient relationship requires the active participation of one physician and one patient, with each of them playing just one role. And in our dealings, I was to be the doctor and Mrs. Magee, the patient. Part of my job as her doctor was to make certain that she really understood her disease, and her job was to learn as much about it as she could. Doctor as teacher; patient as student. Once we established that, we could move on to the more complex relationship that would govern the management of her disease.

Back to basics. "What," I began, "is a seizure?"

She was not interested in my game. "Doctor Klawans. I did not come here to waste my time."

"Indulge me," I replied.

"I've had my complex partial seizures for ten years," she said. "Believe me, I know all about them."

"I don't doubt that, but humor me."

"Doctor Black . . ." she began.

Black was the ex-resident of mine who referred her to me.

"She told me you might be difficult but . . ." she hesitated.

"But what?"

"That I should put up with your idiosyncracies."

"So, put up with me."

"A seizure is a convulsion."

"So, you have convulsions?" I assumed.

"No. Never." She seemed shocked by my conclusion.

"But you said that seizures were convulsions and that you have some sort of seizures."

She looked at me in a new way. Softer. Less hostile. Not friendly, certainly, but more like a student who went to hear a lecture by some famous visiting professor and walked in challenging the lecturer to impress her, and he did just that—for the first time in the student's experience. "I'm not sure exactly. Something goes wrong in the brain and . . ." she shrugged.

We worked it out step by step. The brain is made up of neurons, which send electrical messages back and forth to one another. A seizure is an abnormal electrical message sent out by a group of neurons that are not behaving in their usual, proper way. And this abnormal discharge, in turn, causes some sort of behavior. The exact type of behavior depends upon the precise normal function of these cells. If the cells are responsible for vision, then the seizure starts with bright flashes of light. I gave her other simple examples and then moved on to the subject of temporal lobe seizures, which are now termed *complex partial seizures: Complex* because the behaviors they cause are not simple sensations like flashing lights, but more complicated ones involving thinking, feeling, emotions, and sequential movements. *Partial* because electrically, only part of the brain is firing—the temporal lobe and related structures. Not the entire cerebral cortex: When that happens, the patient has a true convulsion.

And what were her complex partial seizures like?

"I still have them about two or three times a week."

I nodded, fully realizing that she had given me no idea what her seizures were like. I waited.

"The first few were the worst. I just passed out without any warning and fell down and was out for five or ten minutes. And when I woke up, I was so tired and I had a terrible headache."

She had seen neurologist number one then. The CAT scan had been normal. The EEG had shown abnormal electrical discharges from the right temporal lobe. He thought they had been caused by an auto accident she'd been in several years earlier. He put her on Dilantin. The seizures got milder—no more hitting the floor, just brief lapses of consciousness, which the neurologist called absence attacks. Overall, he seemed happy.

On to number two.

Another EEG, another CAT scan. He wasn't as satisfied. His goal was for her to have no seizures at all, not even these minor absence attacks. He was the first one to use the term complex partial seizures. He added Mysoline to her Dilantin, and the absences stopped. Then her spells started.

Another move, and on to neurologist number three.

Complex partial seizures were again the diagnosis, and another EEG was taken. This doctor switched her from Dilantin to Tegretol.

And so the story went, through three more neurologists, several more EEGs, and two more CAT scans.

And now she had come to see me.

"Tell me what your seizures are like."

"They're very short. A minute at the most." She seemed almost disappointed at their present brevity.

Still she had not described them.

I waited.

For the first time, she looked away, gazing down toward the floor.

"All of a sudden, I have this intense warm feeling as if I'm . . . I'm . . . having the most . . . the strongest . . . orgasm and then I am at peace. I've just had an orgasm. And everything is warm and beautiful. That's it."

I should not have been as surprised as I was. Seizures can do almost anything. The particular behavior they cause depends entirely upon which cells and which pathways of the brain were firing. There are cells and pathways that normally relay the physiology of an orgasm into conscious feeling. So why not an orgasmic seizure—a seizure of sexual pleasure? No reason at all.

She was still looking down. I had forced her to describe her seizures, and she was embarrassed by them.

"Do you really want me to treat these seizures? If we're successful, you won't have any more."

She looked up at me and for the first time, she smiled. "Yes," was her answer. Her sex life with her husband was fine. She didn't need to have these orgasms while driving her kids to see the dentist.

Enough said.

We discussed her medicines and made some changes.

Wasn't I going to order another EEG? Or another CAT scan?

No. I knew what she had, and so did she. The question was what we could do to control them.

She got up to leave. "You know," she said, "I have had six other doctors treat my seizures. I've told them all what my seizures were like. You're the only one who ever asked me whether I really want them to be treated."

"I had no choice. One of the major reasons that patients continue to have seizures is their failure to take their medicines. We call that noncompliance. If you don't want them to be controlled, that's your decision, but I don't want to waste my time giving advice you don't want to follow."

"Have you ever had another patient like me?"

"With the same type of seizures?" I asked back.

"Yes."

"No," I admitted. "But I've read about others who had pleasurable seizures."

"In the medical literature?"

"In Dostoyevski."

"Which book?"

"*The Idiot*. His notebooks." I said.

"Prince Myshkin," she said. "I never put it together; I didn't realize." She was amazed. "Dostoyevski was an epileptic. Yet he was a genius."

Here she was, an epileptic herself—for all that term means is that a person has recurrent seizures or epileptic attacks—yet she, too, shared many of our cultural prejudices. "I must reread *The Idiot*."

I didn't have to reacquaint myself with Dostoyevski's works. I had read them before and thought about his epilepsy while reading them. When he was twenty-seven years old, Dostoyevski was accused of sedition and conspiracy against the Russian government. He was placed in solitary confinement for eight months and then sentenced to death by a firing squad. Before the sentence was commuted to prison in Siberia, he was forced to suffer through a mock execution held on a public square of Saint Petersburg before a crowd of several thousand. These shattering events always remained at the heart of both his creative imagination and psychological being. Many of the subsequent events in his life—physical; mental; emotional; medical; and, of course, literary—can be traced back to these experiences. But there is no doubt that he had epilepsy and that many of his supposed psychiatric problems were really neurologic in origin.

How can we be certain? Dostoyevski lived long before the age of EEGs. But it is not the EEG that makes the diagnosis of epilepsy. The EEG can only confirm it. That diagnosis is based primarily upon the patient's history, which must include a series of recurrent episodes that are consistent with seizures. We have Dostoyevski's own history, supplemented by descriptions supplied by his wife, his friends, and even his doctors, which are rounded out by the accounts he wrote of seizures suffered by several of his characters.

When did his seizures start? That's not entirely clear. Dostoyevski himself was convinced that his term in jail and then exile in Siberia resulted in profound behavioral changes, including epilepsy. Undoubtedly, the diagnosis was first made in Siberia. In March 1857, Dostoyevski wrote a letter to a friend in which he confided that the doctor had told him he had epilepsy. This doctor was Major Ermakov, a physician attached to the Seventh Battalion, which was stationed in Siberia. His medical report, written in December 1857, still exists: "Aged about 35, a man of moderate constitution, in 1850, he was struck for the first time by a seizure of epilepsy with the following manifestations: a sudden cry, loss of consciousness, convulsions of the extremities and the face, foam on his lips, stertorous breathing and rapid weak pulse. Duration 15 minutes, followed by general weakness. In 1853, the seizures returned and thereafter seem to have occurred at the end of every month. At this moment Dostoevsky is generally weak and suffers from complete exhaustion and from facial neuralgia as a consequence of an organic disorder of the brain."

His first seizure, however, probably took place in 1846, three years before his arrest and all the events that followed. This episode, described by his friend Grigorowitch, occurred shortly after the completion of his early novel, *Poor People,* which resulted in his first literary recognition. While out walking together, Dostoyevski spotted a funeral procession passing by. He immediately wanted to get away, but before he could, he suffered a severe seizure and had to be carried to the nearest store. He only slowly recovered consciousness. Thus, he clearly had had generalized seizures—convulsions—since 1846.

The writer also had other types of seizures that antedated his imprisonment. Late one night in '46 or '47, a friend saw Dostoyevski's face change dramatically and a frightened look come into his eyes. According to Yarmolinsky, after a few minutes, Dostoyevski asked in a hollow voice: "Where am I?" and ran to the window to get some air. When his host reentered the room, he found Dostoyevski sitting on the windowsill, "his face twisted, his head bent to one side, and his body shaking convulsively." The host then doused him with cold water, but despite this Dostoyevski ran out into the street, with his alarmed host dashing after him. When he caught up with him at the entrance to a hospital which was a couple of blocks away, Dostoyevski had become calmer and allowed himself to be driven home.

Dostoyevski's second wife, Anna Grigorevna, described the first seizure she witnessed, which occurred shortly after the couple was wed in 1867:

> It was the last day of carnival and late in the night after dinner and champagne. Dostoevsky was in a very good mood and telling a funny story to my sister. Suddenly in the middle of a word he stopped, rose from the divan, and began to lean over to my side. I looked with much astonishment at his twisted face, but suddenly came a fearful cry, a cry that had nothing human about it, almost a howl and my husband continued to lean over more and more . . . I put my arms around his shoulders and pushed him with force onto the divan. But you can imagine how great was my astonishment when I saw the unconscious body of my husband sliding from the divan. . . . I kneeled on the floor and kept his head in my lap as long as the convulsions continued. . . . Gradually the convulsions stopped and Dostoevsky regained consciousness; but the first moment he did not know where he was and had lost the control of his tongue; he wanted to say things but mixed up the words, so that it was impossible to understand him.

A friend named Strakov was also present during one of Dostoyevski's seizures and supplied this description: "He stopped awhile as he was searching for a word to say what he meant and he had already opened his mouth. I looked at him with closer attention: I was sure he was going to pronounce some extraordinary sentences; suddenly, from his open lips came a strange, absurd, and protracted noise, and he fell unconscious in the middle of the room."

Dostoyevski may have summed up his condition best. In a letter to his brother, Michael, written in 1855, he confessed, "I have all kinds of seizures."

But what of the seizures that resembled Claudia Magee's: the episodes of pleasure, the periods of ecstasy? Several people have recorded conversations in which Dostoyevski told them that he had ecstatic auras. Auras, the first manifestation of a seizure, are a phenomenon that occurs when only part of the brain is firing and so are perceived by the still-conscious brain and can be recalled afterwards.

Sophia Kovalewski, in her *Childhood Recollections,* reported a conversation that she and her sister had with Dostoyevski in which he told them about what he called his first attack. He had been banished to Siberia when one day he had the unexpected joy of receiving a visit from one of his best friends. It was the night of Easter Eve, and the two friends, though it was late, continued to talk. Like the true Russians they were, they were discussing God. Suddenly, Dostoyevski exclaimed: "God exists, He exists." At the same time a bell from a nearby church began to toll for midnight mass. According to Kovalewski, Dostoyevski went on to say:

> The air was filled with a big noise and I tried to move. I felt the heaven was going down upon the earth and that it had engulfed me. I have really touched God. He came into me myself, yes God exists, I cried, and I don't remember anything else. You all, healthy people . . . can't imagine the happiness which we epileptics feel during the second before our fit. Mohammed, in his Koran, said he had seen Paradise and had gone into it. All these stupid clever men are quite sure that he was a liar and a charlatan. But no, he did not lie, he really had been in Paradise during an attack of epilepsy; he was a victim of this disease like I was. I don't know if this felicity lasts for seconds, hours, or months, but believe me, for all the joys that life may bring, I would not exchange this one.

In one of his letters, Dostoyevski gave this further description of his aura: "During a few moments I feel such a happiness that it is impossible to realize at other times, and other people cannot imagine it. I feel a complete harmony within myself and in the world, and this feeling is so strong and so sweet that for a few seconds of this enjoyment one would readily exchange ten years of one's life—perhaps even one's whole life."

I saw Mrs. Magee next about four weeks later. She was scheduled for a brief follow-up visit of fifteen minutes at the most. After all, not much had to be accomplished and only a few questions had to be answered. Had she had any seizures? No. Was she having any side effects from her new schedule of medications? No. Did she have any questions for me? She did. She wanted to talk about Dostoyevski. She had gone back to his books,

and of course, the one novel she wanted to discuss was *The Idiot*. It was
in that novel that Dostoyevski gave epilepsy the most important role, although as she reminded me, two epileptics had appeared in his earlier
work, *The Lodging Woman*. She had been doing her homework, far better
than I had. I had not reread *The Idiot* for a decade or more, though I did
recall that the character called Prince Myshkin had seizures that resembled
those of Dostoyevski himself. That was why I had suggested the book to
her in the first place.

I did not feel I could discuss a book I hadn't read in over ten years, and
I told her so.

She was not easy to dissuade. She had brought a copy with her and
opened it to a marked place and started to read.

He [the Prince] was thinking of the phase of the onset of his epileptic fits
when they came upon him while awake. In a complete crisis of agony,
stupidity and oppression, it seemed suddenly as if his brain was set on fire,
and his vitality was prodigiously accelerated. During these moments as rapid
as lightning, the impression of the life and the consciousness were in himself
ten times more intense. His spirit and his heart were illuminated by an
immense sense of light; all his emotions, all his doubts, all his anxiety calmed
together to be changed in a sovereign serenity made up of lighted joy, harmony and hope; then, his reason was raised up to the understanding of the
final cause. But these radiant moments were only the prelude to the decisive
stage (this other phase never lasted more than a second) which was immediately followed by the attack; this second was positively beyond his
strength. . . .
    These instants, to define them in one word, were characterized by a
fulguration of the consciousness and by a supreme exaltation of emotional
subjectivity.

As she read, her entire expression changed. She was not alone, was not
some freak of nature. She no longer needed to be ashamed of her spontaneous orgasmic ecstasies. Prince Myshkin had similar episodes; so had the
great Dostoyevski himself. She looked five years younger.

She flipped through to another marked spot and continued reading. "At
this moment, I have foreseen the meaning of this singular expression within
the tenth chapter of the Revelation of St. John, that there should be time
no longer." And Dostoyevski spoke almost in the same terms in his admission to Sophia Kovalewski regarding the case of Mohammed. "Probably
it was of such an instant that the epileptic Mohammed was speaking when
he said that he had visited all the dwelling places of Allah within a shorter
time than it took for his pitcher full of water to empty itself."

Her appointment should have been over ten minutes earlier. But I could not stop her, nor did I wish to. She was learning about her disease and how to cope with it, and the most important part of coping is integrating the disease into your own being and still having a positive self-image. For a year, her self-image had been tarnished. That was no longer the case.

She was done with *The Idiot.* She put the book down, and we discussed it for a while—she as a fellow sufferer looking at its literary and human values, I as a neurologist.

I was an hour behind schedule.

She had more books.

Not *The Lodging Woman,* I hoped. I'd tried to read it once and given up out of sheer boredom. It was *The Demon,* which, she told me, was published after *The Idiot. The Demon* contains one very important passage concerning an ecstatic aura. The aura explains the character of Kirilov and of his strange philosophy of life. In a way, Kirilov seemed to be a personification of certain states of Dostoyevski's mind. She began to read me a dialogue between Kirilov and a character named Chatov. I had no idea who either of them was, but I listened.

Kirilov: "There are some instants, they last 5 or 6 seconds, when you suddenly feel the presence of the eternal harmony, then you have reached it . . . it is a clear indisputable, absolute feeling. You suddenly embrace the entire creation and you say, well, it is like that, it is true. . . . It is not emotion, it is something else; it is felicity; you don't forgive anything because there is nothing more to be forgiven. It is not even love. The most terrible thing is that it is so frightfully clear and such an intense joy at the same time. If it were to last more than these five seconds, the soul would not be able to bear it and would disappear. . . ."

Chatov: "Are you not epileptic?"

Kirilov: "No."

Chatov: "You will be, make no mistake, Kirilov, I have heard it was exactly like the beginning of epilepsy. An epileptic man has fully described to me the sensations which precede his attack; it is exactly like your state, he spoke also of a matter of five seconds and said that it was impossible to tolerate it any longer."

His epilepsy, I reminded her, did not make Dostoyevski a great writer, but it certainly did not prevent it. "But it influenced his art," she protested, "his philosophy, his view of the world."

"Yes, of course," I admitted. "I suppose it would have had to. His seizures were never under control. There were no anticonvulsants then, no Tegretol, no Dilantin. Not even bromides."

"But not negatively," she said. "That's what I've learned. It made his views different. But not worse. After all, Prince Myshkin is Dostoyevski's spokesman, his alter ego. In *The Idiot,* the prince talks about the meaning of the ecstasy preceding his fits and the transformation it produced. 'No matter if my condition is a morbid one, no matter if my exaltation is an abnormal phenomenon, if the instant produced by it, evoked and analysed by me when I recover my health, is a proof that I have reached a superior harmony and beauty, and if this instant brings to me—to an unknown, unbelievable degree—a feeling of plentitude, of fullness, of peace and communion, in a transport of prayer, with the highest synthesis of Life. These cloudy expressions seemed to me perfectly comprehensive, even inadequate.' "

I was now hopelessly behind in my schedule. Mrs. Magee realized she had to leave, but she had one more question. Were there any medical sources she should look up?

There were, even though seizures like Dostoyevski's and Claudia Magee's are admittedly rare. After I gave her a couple of references, she left, and I scrambled to get through the rest of my patients.

The next time I saw her, our discussion focused on the case studies she had tracked down. She started with a 1953 paper written by someone named Subirana who reported two such patients, both of whom had disease involving their left temporal lobes.

The first was a forty-four-year-old man, who for the past eighteen months, had experienced feelings of *"extraordinary beatitude,"* which was "completely out of this world." These increased in frequency to several times daily; while speaking on the telephone twelve days before his visit, he had this feeling, could not speak the words he had intended to, and lost consciousness with a generalized seizure. With the use of anticonvulsants, the seizures stopped, and although the neurological examination was normal, the EEG on two occasions showed *a focus of slow waves* in the left temporal region. An operation over this area revealed a huge, infiltrating malignant tumor. The patient died a few weeks after the operation.

"You don't have a tumor," I hastened to assure her.

She nodded.

"The CAT scans. They're all normal. No tumor."

She smiled. She was convinced.

The second patient, a man aged forty-five, had a father with chronic epilepsy. The subject himself began to have brief periods of impaired consciousness at age fifteen and generalized convulsions at age thirty-five. The convulsions began with a feeling of happiness he was unable to describe;

people appeared different, he "knew what it was like to be in heaven." The sensation, probably lasting but seconds, seemed to go on for hours. He claimed not to mind the convulsions as long as he could enjoy the wonderful feeling. Convulsions came once or twice a month and continued to be generalized, but were accompanied by movement of his head and eyes to the right. The EEG displayed a focus of slow waves and spikes in the left anterior temporal area. With appropriate medication, the major attacks disappeared and the frequency of the seizures of affect lessened, but the content never changed.

"Will you ever be able to control my seizures?"

"Yes," I told her.

"Subirana couldn't."

"That was 1953. We have more weapons."

"I had three spells last week. One while we were out. It was so . . ."

"I am going to put you on a new medication, Depakote," I said. We then talked about it and its side effects.

Before she left, she told me about one other article she had found, by Cirignotta, Todesco, and Lugaresi, published in 1980. The patient's seizures consisted of indescribable subjective symptoms; words were inadequate to express what the patient perceived in those instants. The feelings were so intense that he could not compare it to anything he had previously experienced. While the seizure lasted, all disagreeable feelings, emotions, and thoughts were absent. His mind, his whole being, was pervaded by a sense of total bliss.

What made this case important, I explained to her after she'd finished, was that Cirignotta did prolonged EEG monitoring and demonstrated that this "ecstatic aura" was truly a seizure that began as an abnormal electrical discharge in the patient's right temporal lobe.

"A partial complex seizure," she said. "Just like mine, and just like Fyodor Mikailovich Dostoyevski's."

"But we have many good anticonvulsants," I reminded her.

"Depakote," she said hopefully.

"And others."

Mrs. Magee remained my patient for four years. I never succeeded in getting her completely seizure free, but we did reduce the frequency of her episodes to about one a year, and these generally occurred when she neglected to take all her pills—unintentionally, I'm sure. It's almost impossible to be 100 percent compliant, especially when you haven't had a seizure in months and months.

Author's Note

There are a number of articles on Dostoyevski's epilepsy in the neurologic literature. The following were consulted in writing this article:

1. T. Alajouanine, "Dostoiewski's Epilepsy," *Brain* 86 (1963): 209-18.

2. H. Gastaut, "Fyodor Mikhailovitch Dostoevsky's Involuntary Contribution to the Symptomatology and Prognosis of Epilepsy (William G. Lennox Lecture, 1977), *Epilepsia* 19 (1978): 186-201.

3. P. H. A. Voskukil, "The Epilepsy of F. M. Dostoevsky," *Epilepsia* 24 (1983): 658-67.

Autobiographical and biographical data on Dostoyevski may be found in a variety of sources, including

1. E. Mayne., trans., *Letters of Fyodor Dostoevsky to His Family and Friends* (New York: McGraw-Hill, 1964).

2. James L. Rice, *Dostoevsky and the Healing Art* (Ann Arbor, MI: Ardis, 1985).

3. A. Yarmolinsky, *Dostoevsky, His Life and Art* (London: Arco Publications, 1957).

The article on the EEG documentation of ecstatic seizures is:

F. Cirignotta, C. V. Todesco, and E. Lugaresi, "Temporal Lobe Epilepsy with Ecstatic Seizures (So-called Dostoevsky Epilepsy)," *Epilepsia* 21 (1980): 705-10.

The description given by Dostoyevski's second wife comes from A. G. Dostojevskaya *Herinneringer* (Amsterdam: Arbeiterspers, 1975) and was translated by Voskukil. Ermakov's case history may also be found in Voskukil. Strakov's descriptions were translated by Alajouanine, as were Sophia's reminiscences.

The earliest reference to an ecstatic seizure in the medical literature was written by an Italian physician named Guainerius in about 1440: "I myself have seen a certain choleric youth who said that in his paroxysms he always saw wonderful things, which he most ardently desired to set down in writing for he hoped they would most certainly come in the future. Wherefore the ancients call this disease " 'divination.' " This reference is found in William G. Lennox's *Epilepsy and Related Disorders* (Boston: Little Brown & Co., 1960). These two volumes no longer reflect our scientific knowledge of epilepsy. On the other hand, they bring together a wealth of clinical and historical understanding that our more scientific texts all too often sorely miss. The two cases reported by Dr. A. Subirana are found in *Epilepsia* (1953 [2]: 95-96). They were presented as part of the recorded discussion of the International League Against Epilepsy.

5

The Lizard

It's just a job. Grass grows, birds fly, waves pound the sand. I beat people up.
—Muhammad Ali

I have become a lizard," he began. "A great lizard frozen in place in a dark, cold, strange world. I need the rays of a new sun to heat up this chilled earth, to melt the cement that now encases me, to bring me back to life."

I nodded at him to signify that I had at least some idea of what he was describing to me so graphically. It was probably impossible for anyone who had never experienced the ravages of advanced parkinsonism to understand really how he felt, but I had the advantage of having treated well over a thousand patients who had had Parkinson's disease before I met this man. And although none of them had been able to describe his feelings quite as articulately, I did have some notion as to what having Parkinson's disease really meant.

"And you are to be that sun," he concluded.

His voice was soft, hushed, and never varied in tone. Listening to his vocal characteristics was sufficient evidence on which to make a positive diagnosis, for it had the placed, monotonous quality that is typical of the speech of patients with Parkinson's disease.

His name was Roberto Garcia d'Orta, and he had flown from Madrid to Chicago to see me. He was a tall, thin man in his early sixties, but like most patients with Parkinson's disease, he appeared to be older than his actual age. Not so many years before, he had been an active, vigorous businessman. He was no longer very active or very vigorous. He stood in my office looking at me. His posture was no longer erect, bent forward as he was not by age or worry but by the disease with which he had been wrestling for well over a decade. He had already described both his problem and his need. He had become a lizard in a wintry world, and he was afraid that his own ice age had finally begun. It was then my turn to ask some questions.

"Come," I said. "Sit down. We will talk about your disease."

The vast majority of human maladies are defined either by the exact microscopic changes they cause within specific cells somewhere in the body, that is, their pathology, or by some alterations they produce in the body's chemistry. Making a specific diagnosis of any one of these disorders depends on seeing the cellular changes themselves (through biopsy) or their image (through X ray or other imaging techniques), or by measuring alterations in various chemical indexes (blood tests). Parkinson's disease does not follow this rule. It was originally distinguished from all other neurologic diseases long before its pathology and biochemistry were known. It was described entirely as a clinical entity, a group or set of signs and symptoms that occur together and by doing so make up a specific disease. James Parkinson did not know of any test he could run to prove that a patient had "his" disease. This is still true today: There is no test for Parkinson's disease. No tissue can be biopsied during life to prove the diagnosis, there is nothing to be x-rayed, and no blood test will show up as abnormal. A diagnosis of Parkinson's disease depends upon the physician's skills of observing and understanding. Like beauty and many other human conditions, Parkinson's disease is in the eye of the beholder. And it was up to my eye to behold Roberto Garcia d'Orta's parkinsonism and my ears to hear it and my brain to interpret what I saw and heard.

He turned slowly, moving more like a single piece of granite than a person made of flesh and bones. Neurologists use the term *en bloc,* as a block, to describe this phenomenon. Like his soft monotonous speech, it is an integral feature of parkinsonism. With short, shuffling steps, he moved toward the chair across the desk from me. It took him eight or nine small steps to cross the distance of no more than seven feet. Once there he fell heavily into the chair.

"I have my records with me," he said.

"I would rather start by hearing your story in your own words," I said.

"Can you warm up my world?" he asked again. "Will it be like summer again?"

"That's a great deal to ask in Chicago, in February."

"It is what I need. And not just in February, but even in August and not just in Chicago."

Mr. d'Orta's problem had begun over a decade earlier. He'd been in his early fifties then, what he had considered to be the prime of his life. Perhaps that was what had caused it; perhaps his hubris had angered the gods. No matter. He took a deep breath, sighed, and started again. His voice became a level softer. I had to concentrate to hear his words. The tone never varied—no highs, no lows, no emotional inflections. Flat, soft, hushed, and, at times, halting.

He'd married late in life. His wife was twenty-three years younger. He repeated that figure several times, not in the repetitive rambling of a confused mind but with the genuine concern of a man whose body was failing him far too soon. They had two young children, a boy and a girl. His leather-goods business had been flourishing. Life had been good to him. He'd always worked hard for what he got from life, but still life had been good to him.

Then it happened—not all at once, not suddenly, but slowly, subtly, insidiously, yet perniciously. And inexorably.

What had he first noticed? What had been his first symptom?

A tremor.

Had his tremor been disabling?

He hesitated and thought for a moment. It was a question he had never considered before. "No," he said. "I think not. My hands shake worse when they are doing nothing at all. But," he added, "it was most embarrassing. Even then. I was not ready to be a shaky old man. I still would prefer not to be."

The other problems that make up parkinsonism are not quite so benign and are not as obvious to the patient as is the tremor. They are difficult to perceive and hard to quantify, but they can change a vigorous man into a lizard. Many of these symptoms are collectively called *akinesia* or *bradykinesia,* terms that refer to a number of related symptoms: a marked poverty of spontaneous movements, hesitation in starting to move, and slowness in the execution of voluntary movements. The poverty of movement includes such traits as the frozen or "masked" parkinsonian face. The patient's face lacks both voluntary and emotionally motivated movements. Its features are flattened, and the face itself becomes smoother than normal, so that a frozen or wooden "masked" expression results. Whatever emotional responses occur are slow in developing but can become prolonged, resulting, for example, in a frozen smile. The term "reptilian stare" is often used to describe the characteristic lack of blinking and widely opened eyes gazing out of the motionless facial background, a set of features that truly seems more reptilian than human. A lizard in the eyes of the world.

Mr. d'Orta had gone one step further than the classic "reptilian stare."

He described his entire body as being that of a reptile, and he was accurate; it is not just the face that becomes akinetic in parkinsonism. The entire body shares the same fate. The patient often sits immobile, seldom crossing his legs, folding his arms or displaying any of the wide variety of spontaneous movements seen in normal individuals at rest. The spontaneous movements that we all make constantly but of which we are hardly conscious are no longer made. Patients are rarely aware of this and never complain of it. Their friends and families notice that something is wrong, but what? It is hard to define, hard to describe. The patient looks different—less human, less warm. Perhaps he's merely depressed.

Unfortunately, looking not quite right is one of the minor components of akinesia. Far worse is the fact that the patient has a great deal of difficulty initiating whatever movements he wants to make. The simple task of rising from a chair becomes a trial. The patient has to rock back and forth several times to gain momentum and then push down with his arms merely to get up and walk.

Mr. d'Orta had long had that problem. He had first noticed it about the time his tremor had spread to his left hand. He would drive home from his office, feeling more tired than usual. Perhaps he was working harder. He would finally arrive home, only to discover that he could hardly get out of his car. His body seemed to be frozen into his Alfa Romeo Julietta. He would rock back and forth, slowly at first, until he finally gained enough speed and momentum to be able to swing his legs out of the car. A few more swings, and he could ease the rest of his body through the door.

The next morning when he drove to work, it was better. Not normal, but better. A couple of rocks back and forth, and he was on his way.

His problems did not stop with getting out of the car. Getting up from chairs at home, in restaurants, and at the office and rolling over in bed at night. It was not merely overwork, exhaustion, or fatigue. And he could no longer ignore it.

It was time to see his doctor. That was nine years before he saw me. His doctor sent him to a neurologist. The neurologist talked to him, examined him, and did something James Parkinson had never done; he touched his patient, and in so doing documented the third component of Roberto d'Orta's Parkinson's disease: the rigidity of his muscles. Rigidity is a type of resistance to passive movement. It is felt by a doctor when he or she moves the patient's arm. Normally, there is virtually no resistance to such a maneuver. In Parkinson's disease, the rigid muscle exhibits an irregular jerkiness, as if it were being pulled out over a ratchet or cogwheel. The result is an alternating series of jerks, referred to as *cogwheel rigidity.*

Mr. d'Orta still remembered that examination. The neurologist had moved his arm back and forth several times. Mr. d'Orta himself could see the intermittent jerking or wheeling. "Rigidity," the neurologist had said solemnly. "Cogwheel rigidity."

Mr. d'Orta had never heard that term before, but somehow he knew what it meant. It meant he had a disease, a disease that would affect him for the rest of his life.

The doctor also pushed him suddenly, and he almost fell down.

The story was complete. He had all four of the cardinal problems of Parkinson's disease: tremor, akinesia, rigidity, and abnormal postural fixation. The term *postural fixation* describes the unconscious mechanisms whereby the body maintains its posture. As you walk or sit, your head is held erect not by any conscious willed action but by an unconscious postural control mechanism. In patients with Parkinson's disease, postural fixation of the head is often abnormal. A patient's head tends to fall slowly forward from an upright position, reminiscent of the way a normal person's head falls when he becomes drowsy. So the parkinsonian begins to walk with his head bent forward and his body flexed, more like a monkey than an erect human.

Patients with Parkinson's disease are frequently able to walk quite well and support their bodies against the normal forces of gravity; however, if other forces are added, they may not be able to adjust. A single shove on the chest—which the Spanish neurologist had given Mr. d'Orta—may produce a series of backward steps or retropulsion that the patients cannot prevent. In more severely involved individuals, a similar push may result in the patients falling because of a complete lack of response. This may occur whether or not the patient is expecting to be pushed.

What was happening in Mr. d'Orta's brain? A small group of nerve cells, called the *substantia nigra* or black substance, were unaccountably dying. In fact, most of them had already died. These neurons make a particular chemical called dopamine, which they deliver to another part of the brain, known as the striatum. As the cells of the substantia nigra die, the amount of dopamine they can deliver goes down; it is this deficiency that causes parkinsonism. The striatum helps control movement, and to do that normally, it needs dopamine. Deprived of dopamine, the patient develops tremor, rigidity, slowness, imbalance. In essence—Parkinson's disease.

Mr. d'Orta's neurologist started him on L-dopa. And it worked. He was a new man, almost the same man he had been two years earlier. He still had some tremor at times, and his arms still did not swing normally, but he could get out of a chair, even out of his Alfa Romeo. When his voice became stronger, he discovered that he hadn't realized that it had grown softer. And he could do things more quickly, even those things he had not been aware had slowed down: shaving, buttoning clothes, writing, walking, eating, and one he had never even mentioned to his doctor—making love to his wife.

He was a new man. His face was not frozen. His shoulders weren't stooped. His head no longer fell forward. His feet no longer shuffled as he walked. He was no longer hidden behind a reptilian stare. He no longer looked or felt ten years older than he was.

And, of course, the treatment should have worked. Loss of dopamine causes parkinsonism; L-dopa replaces the lost dopamine. Mr. d'Orta didn't care about that. What he cared about was that it worked. Patients often listen intently as their doctors explain how a medicine works, but they don't really care about its mechanism of action. And I have to admit they are right. Digitalis worked just as well as it does today for the two hundred years that doctors prescribed it without knowing how or why it functioned.

But for Mr. d'Orta the L-dopa did not work forever.

Three years later, he was not quite as strong, not nearly as fast. His voice was weaker. People asked him to speak louder. He shook more. His movements were all slower. He was again staring like a hungry crocodile.

He went back to his neurologist, who increased his dosage of L-dopa, and once again, he grew better—not as much better as he had the first time, and not for as long as three years.

Within six months, his symptoms progressed. He sold his Alfa Romeo and bought a Volvo with high, more upright seats—besides, the Volvo was more fitting for a mature businessman. He rarely went out to eat anymore. His handwriting deteriorated. He quit wearing ties. He rarely spoke on the phone.

So it went: more L-dopa, more deterioration; more L-dopa.

Then the side effects began. Trouble sleeping. Bad dreams. Jerky movements. Sleepiness during the day. He was too young for his body to fail him like this. There had to be an answer.

There was, in the form of a new medicine, bromocriptine.

His neurologist explained the difference in treatment to him. The brain of a patient with Parkinson's disease has lost its dopamine. When a patient takes L-dopa, the brain must convert it into the much-needed dopamine, and yet as the disease progresses, the brain in Parkinson's disease seems to lose this ability as well. As a result, Mr. d'Orta was no longer getting the relief he had once obtained from L-dopa.

Unlike L-dopa, bromocriptine does not have to be converted to dopamine by the brain. It crosses directly into the brain, and the brain reacts as if the drug were the missing dopamine.

Mr. d'Orta began taking bromocriptine, and again improved. Not 100 percent, but he was better for a few more years. Each year, there was progressive disability, with corresponding changes in his medications, balancing the needed improvements with the unwanted side effects. And now he was a slow, frozen lizard searching for the sun. Could I supply the warmth he so desperately needed?

Perhaps; I would make no promises. And what was that ray of light called? Pergolide. It was, I explained, a cousin of bromocriptine. Similar yet different. Some patients who no longer benefit from bromocriptine get better on pergolide. Was he willing to try it? It was still experimental. Its safety was not proved, nor was its value.

He had come to me to seek a new solution; he would try it.

His willingness to take an experimental medication was not the sole criterion for accepting him into our study. The presence of other diseases would exclude him. I ran all the appropriate tests, and aside from Parkinson's disease, he was healthy.

He lived too far away for our usual study, so follow-up would have to be less frequent than usual. Fortunately, we'd already treated over one hundred patients, so we knew what to expect.

Still, his case was unique. I called the chairman of the hospital's Committee on Human Experimentation. Could I treat someone who lived that far away? We negotiated the conditions. Mr. d'Orta had to stay in Chicago until he was on a stable dose of the medication. He had to be seen once every three months by one of the investigators. He had to have a local neurologist I knew and trusted. He had to read and sign the informed-consent form and understand the entire process just as every other patient placed on an experimental drug did.

I told all this to Mr. d'Orta. He, of course, still wanted to try the pergolide. I could not dissuade him, for he had come all that way for something new.

So try it we did.

And it worked. Sping arrived on schedule in Chicago, bringing with it another spring for Roberto Garcia d'Orta. His sun returned from behind the clouds and he could again live the life of a new man. He stayed in Chicago a total of six weeks and then returned to Spain. After that, I saw him once every three months. Sometimes he came to Chicago, sometimes I flew to Madrid, and occasionally we met somewhere in Europe, if I had a meeting to attend.

The pergolide did wonders for the first year. It did fairly well during the second year, and less well the third. Mr. d'Orta had been on it for almost four years when I saw him in Barcelona. I had flown there to participate in a meeting on recent advances in the treatment of Parkinson's disease. He came up from Madrid to see me, and we met in my hotel room.

He had once again become a lizard, and the world was an even colder place than it had been when we had first met. We talked at length. His speech was so quiet I had to strain to hear him. Its slow, monotonous pace was interrupted by brief spurts of words crowded together in a forceful yet soft cascade.

He continued to ask the same questions. Was there anything more I could do? Did I have any new drugs?

I asked him question after question, trying to ferret out some factor that might be contributing to his decline other than the natural progression of his disease. That was undoubtedly the major issue, but it offered little hope to either of us. Before the use of L-dopa, Parkinson's disease decreased the life expectancy by an average of seven years. Today life expectancy is pretty much back to normal, and one can certainly not expect much more from any medication.

Quantity of life, however, is only one factor, for it is the quality of life that must be faced day by day. After many years, Parkinsonian patients begin to develop increased disability, with more rigidity, more akinesia, and worse postural reflexes. Have the treatments for some reason lost their effectiveness? Is the "progression" due to the imperfect nature of our pharmacology? Or is it due to the disease and its inexorable progression?

Probably the latter. L-dopa and the other medications do nothing to combat the advance of the disease. The brain cells, including those that manufacture dopamine, continue to die. Each year, drugs are asked to do more and more. When Roberto first started taking L-dopa, he'd still been working, and it almost turned him back into the vigorous businessman he had once been. He had expected similar results from his medications for the rest of his life, and the medicines had failed him. Or had they? He'd been on L-dopa for fourteen years now, fourteen years of dying brain cells, fourteen years of the progression of his disease.

When he took his first dose of L-dopa, he was far from normal, but he could get out of bed in the morning, brush his teeth, get dressed, eat breakfast, drive to work, work all day, and so on. Now, without L-dopa, he would be not a lizard but a slab of marble—totally immobile and incapable of movement. In fact, had it not been for the very same medications he was certain had failed him, he would probably have died of severe Parkinson's disease several years earlier. I did not tell him any of this. What good would it have done? It would not have changed his needs any and could have served only to decrease his hope, a situation we did not need. And he had such enormous needs.

We talked. There were no other factors, and I had nothing new to offer him.

He nodded all but imperceptibly, but then added, ever so softly, "Implant."

He had read the news, an article in the *New York Times*. A Mexican neurosurgeon named Ignazio Madrazo was doing implants on patients with Parkinson's disease. He was taking a patient's own adrenal gland and putting it into the striatum. The results, he claimed, were miraculous, virtual cures. I was skeptical. After all, the last major medical advance to come out of Mexico had occurred in 1954, when it was announced that laetrile was *the* cure for cancer.

The concept is simple enough. An implant is not the same as a transplant. A transplant consists of taking a healthy organ from a donor and transplanting it into another individual where it replaces that same organ, which is itself in some way diseased: A healthy kidney for a diseased kidney, a healthy liver for a failing liver, new hearts for old.

In an implant, in contrast, cells or tissues are taken from one part of the patient's body and put somewhere else where that tissue is needed. Outside the brain, this is an old technique, and has been used on skin, pieces of bone, and hair. In the brain, however, it's a revolutionary concept.

The brain in Parkinson's disease cannot make dopamine because the brain cells that make this substance have died. So why not implant cells that can make dopamine from elsewhere in the body into the brain? The brain can still respond to dopamine if we can only get it to the right place in the right amounts. So why not implant cells that make dopamine just where the dopamine is needed? Using the patient's own tissue prevents the threat of rejection and does away with the need for immunosuppressive medications. Just a simple operation and the machinery of the brain could be repaired.

There is only one drawback. In human beings, no cells outside the brain make dopamine. But there are cells that make similar chemicals. Along with noradrenaline and adrenaline, dopamine is one of three related substances called catecholamines. Adrenaline is produced by the paired adrenal glands, one of which sits atop each kidney. Because a person needs only a single adrenal gland, one could easily be taken out surgically and put into the brain without endangering the patient's health. Once there and in the right place, it could grow and prosper.

Once the cells grew, they would make adrenaline, and on their way to doing so, they would make some dopamine, as well. Perhaps the dopamine would be enough to help a parkinsonian patient's condition, or perhaps the adrenal cells would be able to fool the brain into reacting as if the adrenaline were dopamine. Why not? The brain responded to bromocriptine and pergolide as if they were dopamine.

That's the theory. The results? It was far too early to tell.

"Im . . . plant," he said once again.

Brain implant—the phrase conjures up images of science fiction. The procedure itself is straightforward and combines two fairly standard operations. A general surgeon removes one of the patient's two adrenal glands. Once it's removed, the surgeon dissects the gland. The adrenal gland has two parts: the outer cortex, which makes steroids and is of no interest in this procedure, and the inner adrenal medulla, which makes adrenaline and dopamine. The surgeon separates the two and cuts the medulla into small slices. In the meantime, the neurosurgeon is preparing the brain to receive the medulla. First, he removes some of the bone over the right frontal lobe of the brain. He then passes an ultrasound probe through the substance of the brain. This probe sends out and receives sound, much like a miniature radar apparatus, which allows the surgeon to locate different structures deep inside the brain. The target is the major fluid-filled cavity (the ventricle) and the striatum just below it. Once he has found the striatum, he removes a small part and then packs the pieces of adrenal medulla into the resulting cavity.

That's it. It's all over, except for the waiting.

"But they've only done it on a few patients," I protested. "We don't really know if it works."

"Im . . . plant," he reiterated.

I shook my head.

"We must wait to see . . ."

He shook his head. "I cannot just sit and do nothing. Like you scientists. My life is winter. Man was not meant to live in Antarctica."

I tried to explain that the scientific community was not just sitting around and doing nothing. They were busily at work. The adrenal gland might not even be the correct tissue. The right tissue should produce dopamine, not adrenaline, which limited a likely source to the brain itself, and more specifically to the dopamine-producing cells of the substantia nigra. But no one had a substantia nigra to spare, especially not a Parkinson's disease patient in whom loss of that specific tissue was the basis of the disease.

There is, however, one controversial source of human substantia nigra dopamine-producing cell. That source is human fetuses. Would this approach work? That was what the scientific community was trying to figure out. In animals, implanted fetal substantia nigra cells are able to grow, and the body does not reject them even though they come from a different animal. Rat fetal substantia cells put into an adult rat grow and prosper. The rat's body does not reject them. Why? It appears that, in some way, the brain, protected as it is by the blood brain barrier (which keeps most foreign toxins and chemicals outside the brain), is itself almost outside the usual immune defense system. Foreign proteins inside the brain do not stimulate the body to produce antibodies.

As a result, the implanted fetal substantia nigra cells mature, reproduce, and produce what substantia nigra cells produce best: dopamine. And that dopamine is enough to overcome the loss of dopamine caused by the destruction of the animals' own substantia nigra.

The procedure works in rats, cats, monkeys, primates.

"In me?" he asked.

We didn't know yet.

Would I do an implant on him?

No. we were not performing them. No one was doing human nigral implants. For now, no one knew even if adrenal implants really work; they don't in monkeys.

That was the last time I saw Roberto. Shortly after I left Spain, he flew to Mexico City.

Apparently the neurosurgical team in Mexico City refused to operate on him. Follow-up would be too difficult. The procedure was not perfected well enough to perform on a patient from so far away. They were operating only on patients who were under sixty years old and had no idea if the surgery would work in older patients. The brain changes with aging, as does the adrenal gland, and these changes could easily have a negative effect on the entire process.

D'Orta did not have anywhere else to turn and pleaded with the doctors, unsuccessfully. But while he was still in Mexico, someone, another patient I think, told Señor d'Orta about another Mexican neurosurgeon. In Juarez. He was not so particular.

Roberto flew to Juarez. The neurosurgeon there greeted him with open arms. As long as Roberto could afford the cost, he'd be happy to do an adrenal implant on him.

"The results?" Roberto asked.

"Very encouraging."

"How often must I come back?"

"Whenever you wish, but your own doctor will take care of you. In Spain."

Were there any dangers?

The neurosurgeon seemed to be insulted by the question. If Señor d'Orta didn't trust him, he could go elsewhere.

There was no elsewhere. "The consent form?" Roberto asked.

"What form?"

Roberto underwent the procedure.

He flew back home two weeks later. He was no better. He was told that it took time for the cells to grow and make the needed chemicals.

How long?

Weeks. Months. Who knew for sure?

Then I received an unexpected call from Roberto's wife. Roberto was dead.

Dead! Why hadn't they called? Why hadn't I been told? What had he died from?

He died, she repeated.

"From what?" I persisted.

"A stroke," she said, and then told me the entire saga.

Roberto was dead. He would never feel another spring. He'd died of a stroke less than a month after an operation on his brain. Had the stroke been a complication of his surgery? It was more than a mere possibility.

Author's Note

Less than one month after Roberto's death, one of our neurosurgeons, Dr. Richard Penn, traveled to Mexico City to study the adrenal implant procedure. We invited Dr. Madrazo to visit us. As far as we could tell, his patients were better. As a center that specializes in the treatment of Parkinson's disease, we felt obligated to study this procedure in our own patients, patients who, like Roberto, had been through all the available experimental medications and had reached the end of their tethers. We chose our subjects carefully, passing over the end-stage, bedridden patients for whom the surgery would be too dangerous, we chose those who still responded to their medicine for part of the day but who, on the whole, remained "off" or frozen in their bodies, lizards existing with only a few hours of sunlight each day.

So far, we have operated on seven patients. Madrazo's subjects did not improve immediately after the operation, nor did ours. Four weeks after surgery, none of them was better. Then they began to notice something. Their amount of down time was decreasing— less "off" and more "on." By week six, the severity of the "off" periods was relenting. There was more sunlight, and they felt less like lizards.

Is it a cure? No, far from it. All our patients are still taking the same medications they were prior to the implants. Whenever we try to lower their dosages, they deteriorate. The original claim for the procedure was that many of the subjects no longer required any medication for their Parkinson's disease. That hasn't been the case with any of our group, nor with any other patients operated on in the United States. Many people have improved; none have been cured. And an implant is not without risk. At Rush, we've been lucky: None of our patients has died. Other U.S. centers have not been as fortunate. Some 10 percent of Madrazo's own patients have died, in most cases from complications directly related to the procedure.

And we don't know how long the improvement lasts. Our first patient received his implant about two years ago. If he or any of the others had been "cured," we'd be doing implants every day of the week. Instead, we are continuing our careful study in selected patients, trying to improve our technique and our results and to learn which individuals we can help the most, and how. Unfortunately, that is the way progress is usually made.

We still do not know why such transplants seem to work at all. The cells of the adrenal gland that we have transplanted into the brain in order to produce dopamine do not survive. Any clinical improvement cannot be related to dopamine production. What then? The best guess is that the cells of the adrenal gland or the cells that make up the inflammatory response that they evoke may be producing a trophic, or growth, factor that stimulates the cells of the brain to develop in ways that overcome Parkinson's disease. This is even more exciting then the production of dopamine, which would only help Parkinsonians, not patients with other degenerative diseases. Nerve-growth factors might help them.

When Madrazo began his work, hundreds of patients flocked to Mexico City to see him. One of these was Muhammad Ali. Ali does not have ordinary Parkinson's disease, but a more widespread involvement of the brain due to the repeated head injuries he suffered as a boxer. The news media were all covering the story. I received a call from CBS. "Would the surgery help Ali?" the reporter asked.

I tried to explain that he had more than just Parkinson's disease.

"So it won't help him?"

"How do I know?" I explained. "I have no idea at all what we are really doing when we put that adrenal gland in the brain."

"So it will help him."

I was getting noplace. This reporter wanted answers, not an education.

"Not as far as we know," I concluded.

Ali never underwent the surgery. All things considered, that was probably the best decision. The possibility does remain that sometime in the not-too-distant future we will be using specific nerve-growth factors in the treatment of many neurological diseases. It is impossible now to know when that time will come and who will be the best candidates.

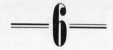

The Flying Scalpels

If it moves, salute it.
If it stands still, pick it up.
If you can't pick it up, paint it.
And don't volunteer for nothing.
—Anonymous soldier

I knew her diagnosis even before my official consultation was requested. In fact, it was only because I had already made the diagnosis that I was finally asked to see her. I was in the army then, stationed at a hospital just outside Washington, D.C. It was spring 1965, and President Johnson was quietly accelerating the Vietnam buildup while promising that the troops would be home for Christmas, although Christmas of which year was never quite clear to me.

One Wednesday afternoon, as I was writing up my consultation on a patient with severe headaches, a woman dressed in a hospital gown walked by me and attracted my attention. Female patients were uncommon in our hospital, except for dependent wives on the obstetrics service. As I watched her proceed down the hall, her legs suddenly jerked out from under her. Fortunately, I had been concentrating on her gait. One of the obligations of being a neurologist is the careful observation and study of patients' gaits. And studying normal gaits—those of individuals who randomly walk by—served to hone my skills.

Both the woman's legs shot out simultaneously, and as far as I could see, their flinging movements were exactly the same. Her arms also jerked out at exactly the same time. While their movements were less violent and less dramatic than those of her legs, they were also paired movements that occurred simultaneously and mirrored each other.

She, of course, fell to the floor, and the movement stopped as quickly as it had started. The single massive jerk, in which her neck also jerked backwards ever so briefly, lasted far less than a second.

She got up immediately without any difficulty. There had been no loss of consciousness, and there was now no obvious weakness in her legs. She patted off her buttocks and continued on down the hall, apparently unperturbed by what had just happened to her.

Myoclonic epilepsy, I said to myself. That young woman had just had a myoclonic seizure. I had never seen one before, which, in and of itself, was not that extraordinary. After all, I'd been a neurologist only for a few years, and only occasionally did neurologists actually see their patients have seizures. Besides, myoclonic seizures are so rare that I had never even seen a patient who had a history of having suffered them. Epilepsy (which simply means the tendency to have seizures) is one of the most common reasons patients are sent to neurologists—1 to 2 percent of the entire population has seizures sometime during life. But of that 1 to 2 percent, fewer than one out of two hundred have myoclonic epilepsy.

Why had I not been asked to see her in consultation? She had a neurologic problem, and I was the only neurologist on the staff. Because she had myoclonic seizures, I *wanted* to see her. I was asked to see every patient in the place with headaches; the least they could do was to share their rare, interesting patients with me.

Myoclonus itself is not rare—far from it, for most of us have myoclonus from time to time. The term *myoclonus,* which is used to characterize a whole host of human conditions, describes a sudden jerk of a muscle or a group of muscles because of a sudden electrical discharge of the nerve cells that control the movement of that particular muscle or muscles. The myoclonus that almost all of us have experienced from time to time is called nocturnal myoclonus. It happens during drowsiness, during the transition from normal wakefulness to normal sleep. All of a sudden, a brief shock-like jerk occurs: The entire body shakes, including the neck, the trunk, and all four extremities. It's over almost before it begins—a single jerk, one shake, and nothing more. You are now more aroused and less drowsy, but you just roll over and drift back to sleep. Unless, of course, your bed partner was awakened by the myoclonic jerk.

Myoclonic seizures are similar, in that they consist of one or two, occasionally three, sudden rapid jerks of the entire body, yet they are in fact a form of epilepsy, a true seizure. But what precisely is a seizure? Seizures are spontaneous uncontrolled movements or other forms of behavior caused by abnormal electrical discharges of the cortex of the brain. All seizures are due to these abnormal discharges. In general, there are two classes of such discharges, focal and generalized. In focal discharges (focal epilepsy), one focus, or part of the brain, fires abnormally and produces a behavior that depends upon the normal function of that area of the brain. If the focus is located in the part of the brain that controls movement (the motor cortex), repetitive muscle jerks are caused. This, then, is called a focal motor seizure. An abnormal discharge in the part of the brain that subserves vision (the visual cortex) results in the sensation of flashing lights (a visual seizure). In the same way, a seizure beginning in the hearing or auditory cortex causes the patient to hear simple sounds (an auditory seizure).

Not all seizures start in one place on the cortex. There are a group of epileptic disorders called the primary generalized epilepsies, in which no one focus initiates the seizures. Instead, both sides of the brain fire abnormally at the same time. Since the two hemispheres of the brain are fairly independent, their simultaneous firing has to be the result of an abnormal discharge that starts deep in the brain and reaches both cerebral hemispheres simultaneously. This is precisely what occurs in myoclonic epilepsy, which is hence considered generalized epilepsy. The other generalized epilepsies are grand mal epilepsy, petit mal epilepsy, and the far rarer disorder called akinetic epilepsy. The symptoms of the four types of seizures differ, since not all cells of the two hemispheres are equally involved in the various seizures. They can be summarized as follows:

1. Grand mal: a generalized motor seizure involving the entire body (the classic convulsion) and accompanied by the loss of consciousness.
2. Petit mal: a brief loss of consciousness (seconds or fewer) with little or no motor component.
3. Myoclonic: sudden generalized jerks of the body (up to three) without an interruption of consciousness.
4. Akinetic: a sudden loss of all muscle tone resulting in a fall without any loss of consciousness.

These are often called the *primary* generalized epilepsies, as opposed to *secondary* generalized epilepsies, in which similar clinical seizures occur secondary to another disease such as a brain tumor.

What I had observed was a myoclonic seizure; the woman therefore had primary myoclonic epilepsy that was due to a seizure discharge that began somewhere deep in the brain. I had to see her in consultation.

But who was she? Who was her doctor?

Her name proved easy to find, for she was the only female patient in that ward, which was a floor reserved for active-duty personnel. Lieutenant Patricia Runnells was a scrub nurse who worked in our operating room. Her doctor was Sam Gordon, an internist and a friend of mine. I walked over to his office and found him free.

"Sam," I said. "You have a great patient."

Sam, who rarely regarded the routine minor illness of basically healthy GIs as exciting, thought I was crazy, "Two ingrown toenails instead of one?"

"I'm not kidding."

"Who?"

"Patricia Runnells."

"She's nuts."

"She is not nuts."

"And believe me, you don't want to get involved."

I told him that that should be my decision, not his, especially since she had a neurologic problem.

"What neurologic problem?"

"Myoclonic epilepsy."

Sam had never even heard of it, or if he had, he hadn't remembered, and he was sure she didn't have it.

"What *does* she have?" I asked him.

He proceeded to tell me her story. She was thirty-five years old and a career nurse in the army. She had been a scrub nurse for five or six years. She was under a lot of pressure. He hesitated.

"Did someone leave some sponges in a patient?"

"It's more serious than that."

"A forceps?" I suggested.

"The CID. And it's no laughing matter."

The CID was the Civilian Investigative Department of the army, which was rarely involved in laughing matters. They were investigating her for alleged lesbian activity. If that accusation proved true, she would be thrown out of the army as a security threat and given a dishonorable discharge. After all, it was 1965.

"What's she going to do? Give the Vietcong our secret method of sewing up a hernia?"

"Don't joke. She is a lesbian, and knows that the investigation is going on."

"I guess she is under pressure," I conceded.

"Last week, in the middle of an operation, she threw a scalpel across the operating room. It's happened three times now, and she's falling down for no reason. She's nuts."

I told him what I had seen.

He was not convinced.

I made a deal with him. He could order an EEG, and if it was abnormal, then I'd see her as an official consultation.

Later that afternoon, we did the EEG. About once every two or three minutes, the normal background electrical activity of the two sides of the brain was interrupted by brief, abnormal high-voltage discharges—precisely what I had thought would be there. They had the classic features of the discharges of the primary generalized epilepsy: They were bilateral (that is, both sides of the brain were involved), simultaneous (the discharges occurred at precisely the same moment on the two sides of the brain), and synchronous (the discharges on the two sides were identical and could be superimposed on each other).

The EEG did not change my diagnosis and did not even influence my thinking. I already knew what she had. It did, however, win over Sam Gordon. He, like all patients and most nonneurologists, didn't understand the role of the EEG in epilepsy. After all, her EEG did show the type of abnormal discharges that we frequently see in epileptics. But epilepsy is not an EEG diagnosis. It is a historical one: depending upon obtaining a history that the patient had some sort of a seizure. A normal EEG cannot change that diagnosis, just as an abnormal EEG cannot create that history for the patient, unless the patient is obliging enough to have a seizure during the EEG. What the EEG does, when you're lucky, is to tell you what kind of electrical abnormality is causing the seizures.

I had seen a myoclonic seizure. Patricia Runnells had myoclonic epilepsy. The EEG confirmed that fact, but it was the observation of the seizure that was critical—that and her history.

I examined Lieutenant Runnells just before I went home that evening. Her history was not precisely what Sam Gordon had told me. It was not all Sam's fault, or hers. She had not given him the same information because he had not asked the right questions. I inquired as carefully as I could about any and all abnormal muscle jerks. They had started about a year earlier as brief mild twitches of her neck and jaw. Her head would move back and her jaw would jut out. A single twitch, as if she was tossing her head. No one thought anything of it, not even her friend. She knew she wasn't intentionally tossing her head back, but she was in good health and happy, so she didn't worry about it.

Over the year, however, the twitches changed. They became more frequent, and by now, she had many per day. They also became more forceful, but not any longer in duration—just a single shock that appeared without warning. They also began to involve more and more muscles: First, just her neck and jaw; then her neck, jaw, and shoulders; then arms; and finally her legs.

The falling had started in the past three weeks.

She was now having about ten to twelve attacks per day. Most involved her head, neck, and arms; two or three involved her legs.

"It's all the pressure," she said.

In a way she was right. Emotional stress can exacerbate seizure disorders. But it wasn't the pressure that caused them.

"The scalpels?" I asked. "Did you throw them during one of your twitches?"

"Yes," she admitted.

I told her what she had. She, too, had never heard of myoclonic epilepsy, but she did know all about epilepsy. Her mother was an epileptic, as were an aunt and her grandfather. The primary generalized epilepsies are, in fact, often hereditary.

She wanted to know what I could do for her.

"A lot," I said. "I can treat your epilepsy so you'll have fewer twitches. Perhaps none."

That she liked.

"And get you a medical discharge."

That she loved.

No CID. No public charges of lesbian activity. No dishonorable discharge.

I started her on Dilantin, and within a week her twitches stopped and her EEG was normal. I talked to Sam Gordon and our commanding officer Colonel Yost, who both agreed: She had epilepsy and should be given a medical discharge.

Pat (she asked me to call her that) stayed with her friend in the Washington area and got a job as an operating room nurse in one of the big private hospitals. I last heard from her about five years ago. She was still on Dilantin, had one or two head tosses a year, and was still working as a scrub nurse. She and her friend were still together.

As far as I know the Vietcong never learned any military secrets from her. Seeing Pat in consultation was the only duty I volunteered for in my two years in the army. Even though volunteering broke an unwritten law, I'm glad I did it.

Author's Note

Myoclonus is one of the most confusing areas of neurology. Virtually all the available reviews are too technical for the nonneurologist. The interested reader may find it worthwhile to look through M. H. Charlton, *Myoclonic Seizures,* Roche Medical Monograph Series (Amsterdam: Excerpta Medica, 1975).

It was while I was in the army that I learned the truth about using EEGs to diagnose epilepsy. I was treating a ten-year-old boy who had petit mal epilepsy with the classic petit mal discharges on his EEG. He was the son of a colonel. He was also a twin. His identical twin brother came into the office with him one day.

Did the twin have spells?

Absolutely not, I was told. One son with epilepsy was bad enough.

Petit mal is hereditary, I thought to myself. If one identical twin has petit mal, the other should.

I talked the father into getting an EEG on his "normal" son.

"Why?"

"To be on the safe side."

The "normal" son's EEG had more abnormal discharges than his brother's. But he had no seizures. And never had had.

What to do? Should I tell the father that this son, too, was not "normal"?

In the end I had to. I had no choice. But all this boy had were some electrical discharges. Not epilepsy. I'm not sure they ever understood the difference. The saying was right— "don't volunteer for nothing." Not even getting an EEG on the twin brother of a patient with epilepsy.

=7=

The Man About Town

I travel not to go anywhere but to go. I travel for travel's sake. The great affair is to move.
— Robert Louis Stevenson, *Travels with a Donkey in the Cévennes*

I never travel without my diary. One should always have something sensational to read in the train.
— Oscar Wilde, *The Importance of Being Earnest*

William Miranda was fifty-six years old when I first examined him. He had not called up to make an appointment, as most new patients do. Nor had his family brought him to my office, as often happens with reluctant neurologic patients. I initially saw him in our emergency room. The police had found him parked in his car about four blocks from the hospital. They had observed him sitting there, staring straight ahead in an apparent daze, for about two hours.

They brought him to the ER about 10:30 in the morning, and he was seen by the internist who covers our ER, then by the psychiatry resident on call, the neurology resident on call, and one of our staff psychiatrists. By the time I was called to see him, it was early afternoon, and his wife was with him.

Mr. Miranda still did not know where he was or how he'd gotten there. Nor did Mrs. Miranda, but she was used to such incidents. In the thirty-five years they had been married, they had occurred at least a dozen times. According to her, the first such episode had taken place some thirty or more years earlier. Willie's brother had recently been killed in an automobile accident, and Willie (the name she always called him by, and which I tried hard to avoid) had been quite depressed. Then, one day without any warning, he walked out of the house. Mrs. Miranda didn't know he was gone until she realized that the front door was open and the car wasn't in the driveway. The next day, he called her from Davenport, Iowa. He had no idea how he got there. He couldn't remember leaving the house or even getting into the car, much less driving all the way to Davenport. He'd awakened out of a fog to find himself parking his car hundreds of miles from home.

His wife attributed it to Willie's "shock" over his brother's death. A psychiatrist had apparently reached a similar conclusion and had placed him on Miltown, the Valium of the early '50s.

Most of the episodes had been pretty much like that first one. They didn't occur often, only once every few years. Sometimes they lasted just an hour or two, and Willie would get only from their home in Waukegan to Milwaukee or Gary, Indiana. The longest lasted well over a day, when he wound up in Fargo, North Dakota.

Mr. Miranda never remembered any details of his travels or of the few hours before they began. He apparently drove reasonably well: he had no accidents or tickets. He never ended up in a ditch or a snowbank. And he never ran out of gas, always remembering to refill the tank as he drove around. Once he even changed a tire. Or at least they thought he did, since when he got home, the spare had replaced the left rear wheel, which was now in the trunk and in need of repair.

Had he changed the tire himself? Or had someone else done it?

He had no idea. But his hands were dirty when he woke up that time—in Conover, Wisconsin—wherever that was.

Once he had three or four episodes and always came back alive and well, the Mirandas stopped worrying about them. They had become just Willie's little trips. Other people had worse problems. They even made a game out of his longer journeys, during which he had a habit of frequently stopping for gas and always charging the bill. As the charge slips came in, the Mirandas would try to reconstruct his itinerary: One of his longer trips had ended in Kenosha, a mere twenty miles from home, but his route had been far from direct:

Waukegan, Illinois

Valparaiso, Indiana

Springfield, Illinois

Fort Wayne, Indiana

Peoria, Illinois

Des Moines, Iowa

Rockford, Illinois

Madison, Wisconsin

Kenosha, Wisconsin

His wife also described many brief episodes of "automatic behavior," during which he appeared indifferent to the environment and performed meaningless tasks, such as repetitively opening and closing windows. In addition, he very occasionally experienced brief flashbacks of a wartime experience. These could be either visual or auditory but in either case always repeated the same sequences. In his early twenties, he had received a medical discharge from the armed forces after sustaining a cerebral concussion.

By now, William Miranda was back to normal, and other than the episode of peculiar behavior that he could not recall, he *was* normal. His neurologic exam was normal, as was his psychiatric assessment and his CAT scan.

Mrs. Miranda was ready to take him home. There was nothing wrong with him. He'd just taken another of his "Little Trips."

I was not so certain. I thought that Mr. Miranda might well have just had a seizure, that his entire trip might have been a part of that seizure, and that medications that help to control seizures might help him. I was well aware that such trips had been described before in other patients with "epilepsy," and that in such patients they had nothing to do with any psychiatric problems. Other neurologists going back over a century have described episodes very similar to those taken by Mr. Miranda. These trips had several striking features:

1. Each traveler carried out complex peculiar behaviors—different from the patient's usual behaviors.
2. Each of them had a complete absence of recall of each entire episode.
3. During their journeys, each traveler retained the ability to respond to sensory/environmental cues.

We did an EEG, which showed seizurelike activity from the left temporal lobe. I put Mr. Miranda on anticonvulsants and, as far as I know, he has not taken another Little Trip since then.

———

Around the turn of the century, the great neuropsychiatrist Emil Kraeplin, who did so much to help define schizophrenia, recognized that compulsive, aimless wandering, accompanied by amnesia, could occur in epileptic patients. He referred to this disorder in epileptics as poriomania (wandering mania). Other authors have used the term *fugue* for any state of altered consciousness associated with the impulse to wander, and this term is now used to cover a variety of trancelike states in patients with or without epilepsy.

Are these poriomanic spells seizures? Are they part of a seizure itself? Or are they the result of something else going wrong in the brain of certain seizure patients?

Most seizures are short—lasting only seconds or minutes. Prolonged episodes of unusual behavior in epileptic patients can be the result of continuous seizure discharges, a state that neurologists call *status epilepticus,* that is, the epileptic state. But in temporal lobe seizure disorders—now called complex partial epilepsy—another mechanism may account for the poriomania. Complex partial seizures that occur repetitively or continuously and result in status epilepticus are rare. Clinical descriptions of those few cases that have been diagnosed describe patients who had prolonged periods of confusion in which they were rarely able to perform complex behaviors. Although most patients had no memory of their episodes, none of them had experienced the ambulatory behavior of poriomania during them.

So ambulation in patients with poriomania is not a part of a seizure itself. But what else could it be? Seizures start suddenly: The electrical activity of the brain goes along normally until the abnormal discharge bursts forth, and with it the abnormal behavior that is the seizure. Seizures end just as abruptly. But the brain cannot return to its normal activity that quickly. The cells that have just been firing away faster and harder than they were ever meant to fire are exhausted. They cannot function as they normally do. It takes time for them to recover. In the patient with a grand mal seizure in which all the cells have been seizing, the seizure is followed by a deep sleep, during which the cells begin to recover from their exhaustion. In other types of seizures, only selected groups of brain cells are firing to the point of exhaustion so that the postseizure (postictal or postevent) state is not one of entire brain collapse or deep sleep, but of loss of function of selected brain functions. Many patients have been described who, during such prolonged postseizure states, had "twilight periods," in which they behaved as if they were in a state somewhere between true consciousness and actual unconsciousness. Such twilight states are frequently characterized by complex activities, often called *automatisms.* This term was devised from the observation that the behaviors often consist of automatic responses to environmental cues. One such patient, a physician, correctly diagnosed and treated a patient with pneumonia during a postseizure state. The physician had no recall of examining the patient, much less of diagnosing and treating him. Another patient who wandered through a forest near her home for several days did not remember this episode. Today, most neurologists who have studied such cases believe that automatic behaviors are due to the slow, irregular recovery of the temporal lobe and related structures from the abnormal electrical discharges (or storm) that make up a seizure, not to the seizure per se.

I believe that William Miranda's Little Trips were periods of prolonged abnormal postseizure behavior. Seizures and postseizure alterations in brain function were what caused him to wander aimlessly around the Middle West. The other, shorter episodes of automatic behavior that his wife described to me always began abruptly. One minute he was normal; the next he was not. During these episodes, he seemed to be indifferent to what was going on around him. He would neither speak nor answer questions. Instead, he would repeatedly perform meaningless tasks: opening and shutting a window, washing his hands over and over again, or taking off his shoes and putting them back on. If his wife spoke to him, he would often reply but always with one- or two-word answers. Never any more.

Once he started on his medication these spells also stopped.

Recently Richard Mayeux and his colleagues from the Department of Neurology of Columbia University described three patients who closely resembled William Miranda. All three ceased their wanderings when their seizures were controlled with drug therapy. When the seizures stopped, the trips disappeared. These results suggest that the trips are a part of the seizures, not just a psychiatric or psychological state in patients who have epilepsy. Medications that stop seizures thus prevent the postseizure states from occurring.

The patient in the neurological literature who most closely resembles William Miranda was not one of Mayeux's three patients, but a Frenchman who lived a century ago and whose disease was diagnosed without benefit of an EEG by Jean Marie Charcot, the father of French neurology. On Tuesdays, in 1887–89, Charcot delivered lectures on general neurology at the Salpetrière, which were transcribed by his students and later published. Some of these have recently been translated by Christopher Goetz, a neurologist at Rush Medical College in Chicago. At the time, Charcot was at the height of his career, and whenever he taught the amphitheater overflowed with students and medical dignitaries.

The Tuesday lectures were impromptu dialogues between the doctor and his patients. Charcot sat on the stage, his profile to the audience and the patient. Footlights and even a spotlight intensified the drama. Slowly and carefully, Charcot would dissect each case history and then, applying neuroanatomic analysis, reach his conclusion. One such lecture involved a patient who had recurrent episodes of amnesia of which he had only fragmented recall. True poriomania. This delivery man had been well until his attacks began at age 36; between episodes, he was normal. The attacks lasted hours or days and were never preceded by a warning sign. Suddenly, in the midst of his delivery tasks, he lost all awareness of his surroundings and walked throughout Paris and the surrounding countryside, interacting appropriately with other people. After awakening, he had partial vivid memories of only moments of these spells.

"In hearing this man's tale," Charcot told his audience,

I wondered what all this meant—what this singular state of unconsciousness really was. All of a sudden, for a few days or few hours, an episode of oblivion invades a man's life. I felt if I could prevent this man from uselessly walking about the streets and through the city, I would be offering him something significant.

From all this information, I believed and I will try to substantiate my opinion, that this man's illness is, in fact, epileptic in origin. I will use the expression "ambulatory automatism," based on descriptions I made in the past of patients who walk about automatically and do not show any external signs that their walking is unconscious.

Charcot was the first professor of neurology and in many ways the father of us all. He was a brilliant teacher and clinician, able to differentiate conditions that had never been described before. His clinical diagnoses were based on the history he obtained and what he observed, not the CAT scan or the EEG or an unending list of numbers generated by some biochemistry lab. He did not need an EEG to know that his patient's poriomania was the result of a prolonged seizure state. All he had to do was talk to the patient and listen to him and he knew. Often that is all that is really necessary, but it has become a skill that fewer and fewer physicians have or use. Why? The usual excuse is the fear that if all the tests aren't done and something goes awry, the patient could sue for malpractice. I don't buy that. That is no excuse for not taking a careful history and analyzing that history before the EEG is ordered. The reverse is easier. It's also more profitable in many cases, and it is what the patient has come to expect.

A patient comes to see me. I talk to him. I watch him. I tell him he has Parkinson's disease. "But you did no tests," he complains in disbelief.

"There are no tests for Parkinson's disease," I try to explain.

The explanation falls on deaf ears. "What about a CAT scan or an MRI scan?"

"They are usually normal in Parkinson's," I tell him as I write out the order, knowing that nothing else will satisfy the patient.

Two weeks later the patient is back in my office. His CAT scan is normal. But now he believes that he has Parkinson's. Why? Ask the patient, not me.

I'm afraid we will never go back to the days when the physician and the patient alike depended on clinical diagnosis. It's too difficult and involves too much time and too much trust. But the diagnosis in a patient like William Miranda should never have to depend on the EEG. He had seizures at odd intervals. Perhaps the EEG would be done at a time when none of the seizure discharges were occurring. Does that mean his episodes weren't seizures? Of course not. But it's easier to just order an EEG. And the patient will believe the results. And so will the lawyers. And the insurance company will pay for it. And the neurologist does it himself and sends the bill. And Mrs. Miranda's cousin had one when she fainted. It's what doctors are supposed to do. And . . . There is no end to the ands.

Author's Note

Charcot's Tuesday lecture on ambulatory automatisms has been published twice:

1. Christopher Goetz, "G. Charcot at the Salpetrière," *Neurology* 37 (1987): 1084-88.

2. Christopher Goetz, *G. Charcot the Clinician* (New York: Raven Press, 1987).

The former is a single essay dealing only with this lesson. It won the Lawrence C. McHenry Award of American Academy of Neurology for excellence in the history of neurology. The latter is Dr. Goetz's translation of a number of such lectures and introduces the reader to the world of late nineteenth-century neurology at its zenith.

There are, to my knowledge, no good discussions of prolonged postictal automatisms that have not been directed at the medical student. The best discussion of modern views of poriomania is that of Richard Mayeux et al. (*Neurology* 29 [1979]: 1616-19). The views of Wilder Penfield and Herbert Jasper, pioneers of the modern approach to epilepsy surgery, are in their monumental work *Epilepsy and the Functional Anatomy of the Human Brain* (Boston: Little, Brown & Co., 1954) and are as vivid and exciting as when they were originally written.

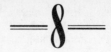

Little Mo

The principal mark of genius is not perfection but originality, the opening of new frontiers.

—Arthur Koestler

The notion of primitive man possessing some inner peace which we civilized people have somehow lost, and need to regain, is a lot of nonsense. Your average New Guinea native lives not only in fear of his enemies, but in terrorstruck dread of the unknown.

—Gordon Linsley

Mo's father had been a high school basketball player. Not an All-American or even an all-state selection, but he'd been both good and lucky—good enough to have been a "star" forward and lucky enough to have played on a team that had competed in the state championship game. His team lost, but no team from his school had ever gone that far, before or since.

When he graduated from high school, Big Mo, who was just six feet tall (a height quite sufficient to play forward in the mid-1940s), went to pharmacy school. He later became a pharmacist, went into business in his old neighborhood, and married his high school sweetheart, who had been the captain of the cheerleaders during their senior year. She had led the cheering during the state basketball championship tournament. She was a real ball of fire who was barely five feet tall.

Life was good to them. The drugstore flourished both as a pharmacy and as a neighborhood landmark—especially during the basketball season. The couple had three children, two girls and then a boy, Edward Morris, Junior, who was immediately dubbed "Little Mo." By age four, it was clear that Little Mo had his father's features and athletic skills and his mother's spirit and enthusiasm. With one exception, this genetic combination was generally thought to be a fortunate arrangement. The one exception was Little Mo's height, for in this he took after his mom, not Big Mo.

At birth, Little Mo was only at the tenth percentile of body length; that is, 90 percent of all newborn boys were longer. By age six, his height had slipped to the fifth percentile. And at nine, he was down to the first percentile, which is short even for a guard. He was no longer just short, he was becoming minuscule. Ninety-nine percent of all boys were taller. By then, not just Big Mo was worried, but his son's pediatrician.

The pediatrician sent Little Mo to be evaluated by an endocrinologist, who discovered that the boy's short stature was due not only to inheritance of his mother's genes but to the fact that his pituitary gland was not producing enough growth hormone. Pituitary growth hormone is one of the main mechanisms by which genes control growth, especially growth of those long bones that determine height. Little Mo had insufficient amounts of growth hormone to reach his hereditary expected height.

In any previous generation he would have gone through life well below the first percentile, like P. T. Barnum's Little Tom Thumb—a pituitary dwarf. But now something could be done. Little Mo could be given the human growth hormone his body was not providing. Growth hormone is manufactured and stored in the pituitary gland. Formerly when patients died and underwent autopsies, their pituitary glands were usually left inside the skull and never even studied. In the sixties, this situation changed. The pituitary glands were collected, and the growth hormone was extracted to be used medically. By the time Little Mo was diagnosed as having an inactive pituitary gland, human growth hormone from autopsies was available to prevent pituitary dwarfism. As far as anyone knew, there were no risks.

Little Mo was given growth hormone, and he grew. He never become tall enough to become a center or even a forward, but at a respectable 5'8", he did play guard in high school. He, too, was the "star" of his team, but the rest of the team was not very good—no state championship tournaments for Little Mo.

In college he switched to baseball, and proved to be a far better shortstop than he'd ever been a guard. In his junior year, he was all-conference. With any real improvement he had a chance to be an all-American—not bad for someone who would have been under four feet tall had it not been for the injections of growth hormone.

Thank God for progress.

When he flew home for Thanksgiving the fall of his senior year, however, he complained of being a little dizzy, but neither he nor his parents thought much of it. By Christmas vacation, he thought he was becoming clumsy and that his balance wasn't quite right. For the first time in years, his father beat him in a game of one-on-one basketball. His mother knew something was wrong.

Over the next year, his balance got progressively worse. He was seen by numerous neurologists, including me, and no one was certain what his problem was. In fact, no one had even a satisfactory idea. His cerebellum, which normally controls unconscious coordination and balance, was deteriorating, and as it did, his ability to perform any sort of activity deteriorated as well. In a little less than a year, he was bedridden and shortly thereafter developed pneumonia and died.

An autopsy was performed. It showed a generalized degeneration of nerve cells throughout the brain. The disintegrating neurons had prominent cavities or vacuoles—a condition sometimes called spongiform degeneration. This condition was first observed in a relatively obscure "degenerative" disease of the brain, a disorder named after the neurologists who first described it—Creutzfeldt-Jakob disease. It usually caused a clinical syndrome similar to Alzheimer's disease.

Little Mo had in fact died of Creutzfeldt-Jakob disease, which rarely begins before age fifty, and never as early as twenty-one. How could this have happened to Little Mo? The moment we saw the vacuoles and made the diagnosis, we all knew the answer.

It had, tragically, been the injections of pituitary growth hormone that brought it on. Creutzfeldt-Jakob disease is now known to be an infectious disease that can be transmitted from patient to patient by tissue contact. But how had Little Mo developed it? He hadn't had an injection of human growth hormone in years.

For nearly a century now, the traditional view of epidemiology has held that all infectious diseases are transmissible, that is, they can be spread from person to person either directly (direct contact) or indirectly (by a secondary host, such as a mosquito for malaria). Once infected, the new host quickly becomes a patient, usually in a matter of days to weeks. Occasionally, it may take months, as it can in rabies, but not years, and certainly not almost a decade.

How could the few injections of human proteins that Little Mo had received when he was ten years old have killed him more than a decade later? The answer to that question involves one of the more interesting stories of modern neurologic investigation, a story that began in Iceland

and New Guinea among sheep and one of the world's last Stone-Age civilizations.

It all started with an Icelandic veterinarian named Bjorn Sigurdsson who had become interested in two separate diseases of Icelandic sheep, visna and scrapie. Visna had first been observed in Iceland in the late 1930s and early 1940s and was thought to be related to the arrival of a flock of sheep from Germany in 1933.

The signs of visna usually began to appear in sheep that were under two years. These early clinical signs included stumbling and lagging behind the rest of the flock. They were followed by paralysis of the hind legs; trembling of the lips; tilting of the head; and, finally, over a period of months, total paralysis. The disease was inexorably progressive, and remissions or survival were never seen. After death, careful pathologic studies demonstrated evidence of inflammatory changes within the brain.

The Icelandic sheep industry was faced with a new disease, the etiology of which was unknown. Was this a new hereditary disease introduced by new genetic material present in the German sheep, an animal analogy to Huntington's disease?

The presence of inflammatory changes in the brain suggested a different answer. Hereditary "degenerative diseases" usually lead to degeneration in the brain—without any evidence of inflammation. Inflammatory changes are the hallmarks of infections. The brains from sheep who died with visna showed inflammation. Had the German flock brought a new infection with them? And if so, what kind of infection?

The search began, and the results were disappointing. The research scientists found no bacteria, no fungi, no parasites.

The outlook for isolating an infectious agent was becoming bleak. All that was left were viruses, but viruses were only known to cause acute diseases, and visna was a slowly progressive, chronic disease.

Was it really infectious? Or was the pathology misleading?

Could it be transmitted from sheep to sheep?

The question was answered in the early 1950s. Parts of a brain of a single sheep that had visna were inoculated into the brains of other, healthy sheep.

At first, nothing happened. The inoculated sheep remained healthy—for one month, for two months, for six months, no infection took this long to develop.

After a year, however, they began to fall sick.

They started stumbling and lagging behind the other sheep. Their illness progressed to trembling and paralysis.

It was visna, and it was infectious. It could be transmitted from animal to animal, but only to sheep. All attempts to transmit visna to other animals have been unsuccessful. In further studies of the experimentally transmitted disease, the sheep appear well during a long incubation period: up to four years can elapse before the signs of paralytic disease develop.

But what caused this disease? What kind of infectious agent? Over the years the Icelandic research workers have conclusively documented that the transmissible agent is a virus.

The German flock had not introduced a bad gene, but a bad virus.

But what about scrapie?

Scrapie was not a new disease in the Icelandic flocks, nor was it limited to Iceland, for it had been recognized by European sheep raisers and veterinarians for over 200 years. It is an invariably fatal condition of adult sheep with a chronic course lasting months or even years. Sheep with scrapie develop progressive ataxia (imbalance, incoordination), tremor, and increased excitability; in the end, they become weak and wasted. Excessive thirst and blindness are also common. The Scottish name *scrapie* refers to a persistent tendency of the sheep to scratch or to rub their bodies against trees or fences, which leads to a characteristic patchiness of wool in the affected sheep.

Initial studies suggested that scrapie was hereditary. Curiously enough, those sheep who later develop scrapie are often unusually well developed as young adults and tend to be kept as breeding stock, thereby increasing the chance for the transmission of a possible genetic trait. Despite the apparent genetic origin of the disease, scientists had transmitted scrapie to other sheep as early as 1936 by injecting extracts of the brain and spinal cord of affected sheep into healthy ones.

The incubation period of scrapie was quite long. It took anywhere from nine months to four years for injected sheep to become ill. Shades of visna.

And as in visna, the only consistent pathologic changes were in the brain and spinal cord. But the findings in scrapie did not indicate any inflammation. There were no pockets of white blood cells, but instead dead neurons filled with tiny vacuoles, a condition sometimes called spongiform (spongelike) degeneration.

Like visna, scrapie was demonstrated to be caused by a virus. Like visna, it is transmissible. Like visna it has a long incubation period. Unlike visna, it did not in any way appear to be an infectious (that is, inflammatory) disease.

In 1954, Bjorn Sigurdsson coined the term *slow viruses* to describe the types of organisms that caused these sheep illnesses. In so doing, he differentiated chronic and slow varieties, two terms that medicine has tended to comingle. The term chronic, he felt, had the connotation not only of a protracted course but of a course that tended to be irregular and unpredictable, such as that seen in tuberculosis, syphilis, and malaria. In contrast, the sheep diseases investigated by Sigurdsson had a rather predictable course that he likened to a "slow-motion picture of the chain of events occurring in the acute infection." He therefore proposed the following criteria for slow infection:

1. A very long initial period of latency lasting from several months to several years.
2. A rather regular protracted course after clinical signs had appeared, usually ending in death.
3. Limitation of the infection to a single species and anatomical lesions in only a single organ or tissue system.

Sigurdsson did add that "these last statements may have to be modified as knowledge increases."

Although these concepts of a "slow" infectious agent leading to death from a "degenerative" brain disease were revolutionary, their relationship, if any, to human disease was unclear. That part of the story began at the opposite end of the world, in New Guinea, where the first true "slow" infection of the human brain was discovered.

Kuru was first described in 1957 after Carlton Gajdusek and Vincent Zigas traveled into the Fore tribal areas of New Guinea and began an intensive study of this peculiar, highly localized disorder. Kuru existed in a mountainous area encompassing about 1,000 square miles and inhabited by approximately 35,000 primitive, Stone-Age Melanesian people. The Fore-speaking natives, numbering about 11,000, had the highest incidence of disease; eight neighboring linguistic groups were less affected. At that time, the natives of this area still lived in small barricaded villages and engaged in warfare, cannibalism, and sorcery. Kuru was the most common cause of death among the Fore, being primarily a disease of women and of boys and girls over age 5; only rarely were men affected. More than 1,400 deaths from kuru were recorded during the first 7 years of the study. Since kuru was thought by the natives to result from sorcery, ritual killing of adult male sorcerers added a secondary form of kuru-related mortality that partially compensated for the severe overabundance of men in a population in which kuru had made women scarce.

The disease starts insidiously with tremulousness of the head and mild difficulty with balance. The Fore people were clearly more astute at making an early diagnosis than was the Western physician. A woman in late pregnancy who was unable to walk easily across a narrow tree trunk bridging a gorge knew she would die of kuru. The physicians examined her and thought she was normal. In less than one year, she was dead. The mild imbalance progresses into frank ataxia (severe imbalance) that follows a relentless course until the patient is unable to walk and finally is unable to make the slightest movement without wild tremors. Slurred speech develops, leading finally to the inability to speak. Although relatives feed the sufferers, difficulty swallowing eventually leads to starvation. The disease progresses for three to six months until death results from starvation, infection, aspiration, or accidental rolling into the fire within the hut. Extensive laboratory examinations of the patients and their fellow villagers failed to show any consistent abnormalities among patients with kuru, and the spinal fluid was found to be normal (that is, no signs of infection were detected).

Pathological abnormalities in kuru are limited to the central nervous system. On visual inspection, the brain appears to be normal, but microscopic examination shows a severe loss of neurons associated with vacuolization of the surviving cells. Again, the results suggested a degenerative disease, not an infection—a spongiform degeneration.

Within two years, Dr. William Hadlow, a veterinarian working with scrapie, pointed out some remarkable similarities between scrapie and kuru in a letter to the editor of *Lancet*. He noted that the epidemiology of the two disorders was similar. Each disease was rampant within a confined population, that is, a flock or a tribe. He further noted that members became sick months or even years after leaving the flock or tribe and that the disease was introduced into neighboring population groups—by intermarriage, in the case of kuru, or by importation of a ewe or ram, in the case of scrapie. Furthermore, the genetic, toxic, and other hypotheses of causation had been extensively investigated without revealing any positive results. The clinical disease itself was also similar. Both kuru and scrapie had insidious courses, manifested primarily by staggering, and both led to death in three to six months. Normal spinal fluid was found in both disorders. And most important, the pathological changes were virtually indistinguishable—neuronal degeneration, with vacuolization. Since scrapie had been transmitted by inoculation and was therefore thought to be infectious, Hadlow suggested that kuru might also be a transmissible disorder and that studies in primates should be undertaken to test this hypothesis.

Following these suggestions, Gajdusek and Clarence Gibbs inoculated chimpanzees with kuru material with astonishing results. All the eight chimpanzees that were originally inoculated with kuru material developed ataxia following an incubation period of eighteen months to four years. The ataxia and difficulty of movement worsened steadily over a four- to six-month period, leading to a moribund state before the animals were finally sacrificed.

Neurologists who have had the opportunity to examine both Fore tribal patients with kuru and chimpanzees inoculated with material from kuru brains have noted the striking clinical similarities between these two groups in both the early and late stages of the disease. Gajdusek and his associates also reproduced the disease in a second "generation" of chimpanzees by inoculating the brain suspensions of affected chimpanzees. The neuropathological findings in the chimpanzees are similar to those in humans, namely, spongiform degeneration.

This work, which culminated in the description of the virus itself, eventually led to a Nobel Prize in medicine for Gadjusek.

The bridge had been gapped. A "degenerative" disease in humans (kuru) had been proved to be "infectious." This was a revolutionary concept. Degenerative diseases were regarded as chronic illnesses of deterioration and were therefore neither treatable nor preventable. A viral disease, in contrast, is infectious, and, as such, could perhaps be prevented by a vaccination. And maybe even treated.

But how did members of the Fore tribe become infected? The mechanism was first suggested by Dr. Robert Gasse, a social anthropologist who lived among the Fore people. Gasse collected evidence that ritual cannibalism was first taken up by the Fore tribe about 60 years earlier, with kuru first appearing about a decade after that. Medical investigators had been told by the Fore that kuru had been present for many generations and assumed that it antedated cannibalism and was probably hereditary. It was an anthropologist who understood that "many" had a different meaning for the Fore people, who still lived in the old Stone Age, than it did for their physician: The Fore counted "one, two, many." Furthermore, cannibalism was practiced primarily by the women, and, in most cases, only the women ate brain tissue from their dead relatives or friends. Women, however, shared these treats with their children, so there is a relationship between the incidence of kuru and the ages and sexes of Fores who cannibalized kuru victims. Since the body was consumed with minimal cooking, transmission of an infectious agent would be possible. This mode of transmission could also explain the presence but lower incidence of kuru in surrounding tribes, since the neighboring peoples, who were also cannibals, refrained from eating known kuru victims. Cannibalism has been actively suppressed in the Fore area since it came under control and study in the 1950s, and in recent years, there has been a striking decline of the incidence of kuru, most dramatic among the children, in whom the disease quickly disappeared. A degenerative disease was found to be a viral disease, which was eradicated by effective disease control.

What does all this have to do with Little Mo?

In some ways, Creutzfeldt-Jakob disease is the opposite of kuru. It is not a disease that occurs commonly in a peculiar, isolated population but, rather, is a rare illness that strikes every once in a while throughout the "civilized" world. It presents in older adults as a progressive dementia reminiscent of Alzheimer's disease, but it is more rapidly progressive and is often (usually) associated with lighteninglike muscle jerks (myoclonus). Occasionally, it presents as progressive imbalance or ataxia. The great choreographer George Balanchine died of this form of Creutzfeldt-Jakob disease.

There is, however, one similarity between Creutzfeldt-Jakob disease and kuru—their pathology, which involves the loss of neurons with vacuolization. The authors of the first description of the pathology of kuru had recognized this resemblance. Immediately after his success with kuru, Gadjusek and his co-workers carried out comparable research on Creutzfeldt-Jakob disease with similar results. Creutzfeldt-Jakob disease was transmitted to a chimpanzee. Thirteen months after intracerebral inoculation of cerebral biopsy tissue from a patient, the chimpanzee developed ataxia, tremor, and intermittent jerking of the extremities (myoclonus). At autopsy, pathologic features that are typical of Creutzfeldt-Jakob disease were found. Further studies showed that the disease could be transmitted from chimpanzee to chimpanzee.

Thus, Creutzfeldt-Jakob disease is transmissible and infectious.

It can be spread to chimpanzees and to humans. A patient who received a cornea from a patient with the disease developed it one year later. A neurosurgeon who inadvertently cut his hand while doing a brain biopsy on a patient with the disease developed dementia and died in fewer than two years.

Brain tissue can be infectious. It can spread Creutzfeldt-Jakob disease. And the pituitary gland develops from the brain. Could it carry the disease?

Of course. If the cornea can, the pituitary and its extracts can. The virus of Creutzfeldt-Jakob disease is "sticky" and tends to attach to various proteins, one of which is human growth hormone.

Little Mo was one of over 10,000 Americans who received growth hormone. How many of these patients developed Creutzfeldt-Jakob disease? Or might yet develop it?

Creutzfeldt-Jakob disease is a rare disorder. About 150 people die of it in the United States each year. Only a few of the batches of growth hormone could possibly have been contaminated by the virus. So far, only a few cases have come to light, and it appears unlikely that many new cases will appear. The method used to obtain human growth hormone was switched in the late seventies to a "virus-proof" procedure, and now human growth hormone is no longer used. Now bacteria have been trained to produce the exact same molecule—a molecule that is free from any possibility of viral contamination.

Kuru no longer exists except in laboratory animals, kept alive by sequential passage from animal to animal. But no one in New Guinea gets kuru or dies of it. It was eliminated by eliminating the means by which it was spread. No cannibalism, no kuru.

Scrapie and visna were eliminated, by isolating all infected animals and preventing the contamination of other sheep.

Visna is caused by a virus from the same family as the AIDS virus. The analogy is obvious. Unfortunately, it is far easier to regulate the behavior of sheep than of humans. It is possible that AIDS will be controlled by a vaccine or by treatment. But those may take years or decades to develop. The disease can be eliminated by controlling the spread of the infection. The choice is ours.

Author's Note

The spread of Creutzfeldt-Jakob disease by human injections of human growth hormone has been the subject of many recent articles. The following put it all in perspective:

1. E. B. Rappoport, "Iatrogenic Creutzfeldt-Jakob Disease," *Neurology* 37 (1987): 1520–22.
2. P. D. Brown, "Human Growth Hormone Therapy and Creutzfeldt-Jakob Disease: A Drama in 3 Acts," *Pediatrics* 81 (1988): 85–99.
3. P. D. Brown, "The Decline and Fall of Creutzfeldt-Jakob Disease Associated with Human Growth Hormone Therapy," *Neurology* 38 (1988): 1135–36.

The story of kuru and other "slow" virus infections can be found in R. W. Hornabrook, "Slow Virus Infections of the Central Nervous System," *Handbook of Clinical Neurology 34* (Amsterdam: Elsevier, 1988), 275–91.

Sigurdsson's classic definition of slow viruses appeared first in "Rida, A Chronic Encephalitis in Sheep," *British Veterinary Journal* 110 (1954): 341–47.

Creutzfeldt-Jakob disease used to be known as Jakob-Creutzfeldt disease. Creutzfeldt described the disease first, but Jakob described five patients, while Creutzfeldt described only one. A careful rereading of these papers raises the distinct probability that the one patient Creutzfeldt studied did not have the disease. Perhaps it should be called just Jakob disease.

9

Making the Playoffs

About once a month, until the age of 70, George Bernard Shaw suffered a devastating headache which lasted for a day. One afternoon, after recovering from an attack, he was introduced to Nansen and asked the famous Arctic explorer whether he had ever discovered a headache cure. "No," said Nansen with a look of amazement.

"Have you ever tried to find a cure for headaches?"

"No."

"Well, that is a most astonishing thing!" exclaimed Shaw. "You have spent your life in trying to discover the North Pole, which nobody on earth cares tuppence about, and you have never attempted to discover a cure for the headache, which every living person is crying aloud for."

—William G. Lennox

Ron Pringel was not the best resident I ever trained. To start with, he was not the brightest. I take no credit for the brightness of my residents: Whatever has or has not made them particularly bright happened long before they ever walked into my office. The same is true of their work habits, and Ron was not a particularly hard worker. He did his share and went home. No less, but never more. His knowledge of medicine was average. He had not gone to one of the better medical schools, and his exposure to neurology there had been limited. But he had come to our department to learn neurology, and that much we could, and would, teach him.

A neurology residency lasts three years. Ron was one of four first-year residents. Although I never try to compare them, it's impossible not to as you go from bedside to bedside, from consultation to consultation, from one sick patient to the next. During the first year, Ron had a mixed score card:

Basic intelligence: second

Basic knowledge of medicine: third

Basic knowledge of neurology: second

Work habits: third

Determination to succeed: first (tied with one other)

Street smarts: first—far and away

I also grew to like him personally and knew that we would remain friends long after his residency ended. No matter where he went, he would not disappear from my life. And he didn't.

As soon as he completed his residency, Ron moved to California—Los Angeles to be exact—and went into private practice. He opened his office on July 1. He called me about a patient on July 2. And about once a week afterward during the course of that summer. Most of the calls were to have his old boss tell him he was doing the right thing. Occasionally, he asked for advice.

On September 23, he asked for help with an acute neurologic emergency. The problem was not the diagnosis—he had identified the patient's illness—nor the treatment—he knew all the appropriate treatment options for the disease.

What was the problem, then?

It was the patient. He was a star pitcher for the Dodgers. It was not clear to me what difference that made. Ballplayers have the same neurologic problems as everyone else, and the same needs. And you treat them in the same way. Besides, Ron was not a Dodger fan, or he hadn't been in June when he'd left Chicago. He'd grown up watching the Yankees—Mickey Mantle, Yogi Berra, and Roger Maris. He had a baseball inscribed to him by a perfect-game pitcher, Don Larsen. What did he care about the Dodgers?

"I converted," he admitted.

Heresy. I lived in Minneapolis for a year, and never once considered deserting my White Sox. So what was the problem?

"He has headaches."

"All God's children have headaches. What's the big deal?"

"He has cluster headaches. He hasn't played in two weeks. And the playoffs start in ten days. I have to make sure he plays."

"Why? Did you bet on the playoffs?"

"No. Not for him. For me. For my career here in L.A."

I was beginning to understand. "Tell me about his headaches."

They had begun a little over a month before. Each one lasted about an hour and a half. The pitcher had four to six each day, which meant that each week, six to nine hours of excruciating pain would come and go without warning and leave the patient physically and emotionally a wreck.

No wonder he wasn't pitching. And if the headaches continued, he wouldn't pitch in the playoffs, or the World Series—if Ron's diagnosis was correct. In headaches, diagnosis is all, for the diagnosis defines both the prognosis and the treatment. And the diagnosis is not based on any tests. Headache clinics may do all kinds of testing, but it rarely helps the patient. The diagnosis is based on history.

"What are the headaches like?" I asked Ron.

"I tape recorded his own description. I'll play it for you."

In a moment, I was listening to an all-star pitcher.

"The first one came on about three in the morning. I'd beaten the Cubs that night. I'd pitched good. Not my best, but I went eight innings. And I had them Cubs eating out of my hand most of the time. I was only in real trouble twice and hell, the shortstop . . ."

"Tell us about your headache," Ron's voice said, attempting to focus the narrative. I wondered what the shortstop had done.

"I felt real good after the game. So we went out to eat. Me and June. We've been together since May. Almost as long as we've been in first place. She's my good luck charm."

Ron cleared his throat.

"I was feeling really up. Full of energy. We had a bottle of champagne to celebrate. I don't usually drink nothing. But this was an occasion. It had been my eighteenth win. That's one more than I won all last year. I was seventeen and eleven last year. So far now, I'm . . ."

Another cough.

"Oh . . . year. Then we drove home. She sort of lives at my place. Except when we're on the road. I got into bed and was waiting when . . . whacko! It hits me."

This time he stopped himself, as if he had given a description. So far, he had supplied only a few facts: There was a sudden onset of something, which was preceded by a feeling of elation and the consumption of alcohol. But the sudden onset of what?

Ron had more or less asked thè same question.

"Pain," the pitcher replied.

"Where?"

"In my head."

"Can you be more specific?" Ron asked. It is often difficult for patients to describe pain. Pain is pain; it hurts. Delineating its attributes—such as character, location, and duration—is often difficult, but not in true cluster headaches. The pain of a cluster headache is usually so severe, so dramatic, so different that the patient recalls it with anguished specificity.

The pitcher recalled the details quite clearly. The pain had hit him like a jolt of lightning, a sudden stab with a sharp knife, right into his left eye, and went on in continuous jolts.

"I felt just like Herb Score," he explained. I knew just what he meant. Score had been a brilliant left-handed pitcher for the Cleveland Indians, one of the best pitchers in baseball, a twenty-game winner, the strikeout king. He was headed for the Hall of Fame, until one evening in Cleveland. Score wore glasses. He threw a fast ball to Gil McDougald. McDougald hit it, and smashed the ball straight into Score's face, sending glass into his eye. That, for all practical purposes, was the end of Score's career.

Every pitcher's nightmare. And there it was, happening to Ron's patient in his own bed.

From his eye, the pain spread—to his left temple, to his left forehead, to his left nostril, to his left jaw, and especially to his teeth, the molars. He sat up in bed. He felt closed in. His nose was stuffed up.

"Your entire nose?" Ron asked him.

No. Just the left side. It was completely stuffed up, but it was running. I was sure if I could sneeze I would feel better, but I couldn't. I tried and tried, but nothing happened.

The jabs just kept coming. I went into the bathroom and looked in the mirror. My face didn't look like me no more. I'm out in the sun a lot. I've got a good tan, especially on my face. But not then. I looked pale. And also flushed. Pale on the right. Red on the left. My left eyelid was drooping. And the left eye was pink. It's bloodshot. I hadn't drunk that much. And the right eye's okay.

I ran the cold water and put a cold washcloth over my eye, but that don't do no good. I've got to keep moving. I start walking, pacing. Like a nervous manager. It doesn't help. Nothing helps. It's like the pain will never end. And it's only been going on for ten minutes.

The pain is incredible. Suddenly I'm in a fury. I picked up a chair high over my head and smashed it to the floor. I doubled my fist and smashed the wall over and over again. The pain doesn't go away.

The episode lasted fifty-five minutes more, and when it was over, his head felt fine. Only then did he notice the dull ache of his right hand—his pitching hand. It had been caused by smashing the wall: his knuckles were raw.

All the subsequent headaches had been just like that first one: sudden onset; localized severe pain, always in the exact same place; brief duration—fewer than two hours; and sudden resolution. All of them were accompanied by the same associated symptoms: nasal congestion, running nose on the side of the pain (unilateral, ipsilateral rhinorrhea, to be technical), unilateral bloodshot eye with tearing (lacrimation). He had four to six attacks each day. Day in, day out. Night in, night out.

The diagnosis was obvious. The Dodger star right-hander had a sore right hand and cluster headaches. Cluster headaches are not a new disease. They date at least as far back as the German neurologist Moritz Heinrich Romberg, who published the first clinical textbook of neurology in 1840. In that work, Romberg recounted the case of a patient with one-sided head pains associated with ipsilateral lacrimation and conjunctival redness. Since then, the same syndrome has been described many times under many names, varying from eponyms (Bing's headache, Horton's cephalalgia) and descriptive titles (red migraine, cluster headache) to others (such as greater superficial petrosal neuralgia) whose specific meaning is often unclear even to neurologists. The name *cluster headache* was first used in 1952 by E. C. Kunkle, an American neurologist who noted the distinctive clustering of the headaches in his series of thirty patients. Most patients have these headaches in clusters. A typical cluster is characterized by one or more headaches per day, and the episodes may recur for from a couple of weeks to a couple of months, but rarely longer. Between the clusters, there are no headaches.

What causes such headaches?

We have no idea. We don't know what causes the tendency to have a cluster of headaches, what brings on the cluster, or why a particular headache starts when it does or why it just as suddenly stops. Dilation or swelling of blood vessels plays some role. Swelling of the temporal artery and increased blood flow cause the conjuctival injection, nasal stuffiness, lacrimation, rhinorrhea, and flushing. The dilation of arteries also causes the pain.

But why does this all happen? The mechanism remains unclear, although individual episodes or clusters are sometimes triggered by exposure to substances that can act directly on blood vessels, including alcohol. Alcohol, including the alcohol in champagne, can and does dilate blood vessels, and our pitcher had champagne before his headache erupted.

"Your diagnosis is correct," I said.

"I know that. So, what should I do?"

"Treat him."

"He's already been on everything, and nothing has helped. And he has to be ready to pitch in ten days."

"Too bad he hasn't had clusters before."

"But he has."

"How many times?"

"Twice. Is that important?"

"It could be. In many patients, the clusters always last the same amount of time. I had one guy whose clusters always lasted forty-five days. If his first two clusters were about the same duration, then at least you can make a prediction."

"What if they lasted sixty days?"

"Bet on the Milwaukee Braves," I replied.

"They're in Atlanta now."

"What are the Milwaukee Braves doing in Atlanta?" I asked. "They just left Boston."

Ron hung up.

The next I heard about the pitcher was when I watched him win two games in the World Series. I had been out of the country for the playoffs. After the series, I called Ron. What had happened?

Ron had gotten further details of the previous two series of headaches. Each had lasted exactly forty days and forty nights. Precisely forty days.

And Ron had seen the pitcher and called me on day thirty of the third cluster.

"So you told him they'd go away in ten days."

"Not quite."

"Not quite?"

"Well, no. I handed out a complicated schedule of vitamins, weak tranquilizers, useless vasodilators. Lots of pills that couldn't possibly hurt him. But the schedule was very long and very detailed—different pills at different times each day. And I told him that if he followed it, the headaches would be gone in ten days. I also told the owner."

"And it worked?"

"Of course. He followed my schedule. And the headaches were gone in ten days."

"They would have been no matter what he did."

"I know that," Ron said. "And you know that, but no one else knows that."

He was right about that.

"And I never lied."

That was true. He had given the patient a set of instructions and told him that if he did as ordered, he would be well in ten days. Ron had never said that if the pitcher didn't comply, the headaches would go away anyway. He just never mentioned the prognosis.

Today Ron has a very successful practice and treats a lot of professional athletes. And I have a baseball signed by a pitcher who has cluster headaches. I'd rather have the one signed by Don Larsen, even if he did pitch for the Yankees.

I have visited Ron several times over the years. He has sent me patients. I send him patients. Whenever I'm asked to recommend a neurologist in L.A., I recommend him. I am still hesitant to compare my residents, but once they are out in the world and I have to chose someone to take care of a patient of mine all of that hesitancy disappears. Only the best is good enough. And Ron is one of the best. His "street smarts" have developed into an instinctive clinical acumen that I respect. His "successful" treatment of this pitcher's cluster headaches probably did more than his clinical skills to develop his practice. True, it was more show business than medicine. But was it all show business? Patients have more faith in medications than predictions. And baseball players are often very superstitious. Perhaps what Ron did was good medicine, too. Perhaps it helped to assure that history would repeat itself. We'll never know. But it was sure good show business. And what else do you need in L.A.?

Author's Note

The only authorative work on cluster headaches is *Cluster Headache* by Lee Kudrow (New York: Oxford University Press, 1980).

In many respects, modern neurology began with Moritz Heinrich Romberg (1795–1873), who first brought order and system to the study of neurologic disease. Romberg was born in Meiningen and studied medicine at the University of Berlin. Following his graduation in 1817, the 22-year-old Romberg decided to devote his life to the study of diseases of the nervous system. To pursue this aim, he went to Vienna, where one of his teachers was John Peter Frank (1745–1821). Frank was one of the great pioneers of public health and had written a major treatise on the pathology of the spinal cord.

As with all great clinicians, patients and their afflictions were the major influences on the work of Romberg. In the introduction to his textbook, Romberg described their significance:

> I availed myself of the opportunities afforded in our large hospital, la Charite of examining all the patients labouring under cerebral disease. . . . I had ex-

tensive opportunities of examining patients during life and after death. For twenty-eight years I was physician to one of the largest unions in Berlin, in which on the average, 200 patients presented themselves annually; among them were a large number of nervous patients, most of whom I presented to my pupils in the lectures which I delivered in the University since 1834. Some of the results of these investigations have been laid down in my academical Essays.

The influence of his patients, combined with his deep understanding of basic neurologic science, resulted in his revolutionary *Lehrbuch der Nervenkrankheiten des Menschen* [textbook of human nervous diseases], which appeared in segments between 1840 and 1846. This textbook provided the first systematic approach to clinical neurology and included the first description of cluster headaches.

The anecdote involving George Bernard Shaw and Nansen appears in Lennox's *Epilepsy and Related Disorders* (Boston: Little, Brown & Co., 1960).

=10=

The Twenty-Five-Cent Cure,
or Cheap at Half the Price

I'm tired of all this nonsense about beauty being only skin deep. That's deep enough.
What do you want—an adorable pancreas?

—Jean Kerr

Movement disorders, like beauty, are in the eye of the beholder. This simile is not just a bad pun. While the major diseases that constitute the field of movement disorders are primarily diagnosed on the basis of what the skilled observer sees, complemented by the patient's history, the decisive factor is what the observer discerns. There is no diagnostic test that proves that a patient has chorea or tics or Parkinson's disease or dystonia. The list goes on and on. The diagnosis of any of these conditions is made because the movements the patient manifests fit one of the respective categories of disorders. And the ability of the physician to categorize (diagnose) these diseases depends upon the skill of his eye. And that is much like appreciating beauty. Today, Monet's Water Lilies represent a form of beauty. So do Van Gogh's Sunflowers. That was not always so; we have been trained to appreciate the beauty in them. In much the same way, I have been trained to see the diseases that cause the abnormal jerks and twitches that patients bring with them to my office.

Joseph C. Martin, Ph.D., had come from Arizona to Chicago to let me have a look at his problem. Joseph Martin had a movement disorder. In a broad sense his history was the same as that of most patients with these disorders. He had had the abnormal movements for some time, and they were getting worse. His doctor had tried him on a series of medications without much benefit and did not know what else to do for him. That is not intended as a criticism of the physician, who was a general practitioner and had received little training in neurology and none in movement disorders per se. Yet the GP had correctly diagnosed his patient as having some sort of movement disorder and suggested that he either see someone who specialized in movement disorders or give up.

Joseph Martin was not willing to give up.

Patients are often bothered that I diagnose their disease by merely looking at them. I should be ordering tests and poring over X rays and CAT scans and what have you. Joseph Martin understood that in my field, those procedures rarely help. His doctor had already explained all that to him in great detail. Joseph Martin, Ph.D., had no trouble with such a concept. He had a doctorate in philosophy, which he had taught for over forty years, retiring two years earlier when he reached age seventy.

His abnormal movement had begun some eight years before his visit to me. Whenever he was writing, his fingers would begin to cramp and curl under. If he stopped, the cramp stopped, his fingers uncurled all by themselves. At first, this cramping occurred only after he had been writing for several minutes. So every few minutes, he would put his pen aside and wait for the cramp to go away.

It was no big deal, more an aggravation than a disability, but it did cause some problem in writing out his lectures.

He told his wife about the cramps. That year, she bought him a new pen for Christmas—a nice, thin Cross pen that she was convinced would be much easier to use than the throwaway pens he normally wrote with.

The Cross pen didn't help, and, although he suspected that it made his problem worse, he used it. It was a gift from his wife.

Over the years, his cramp grew more pronounced. Less and less effort was needed to elicit it, until it started as soon as he picked up the pen. And it was no longer limited to his fingers. The cramp still began with a forceful curling of the fingers, but now as he wrote, the wrist bent downward and rotated, and his elbow spontaneously lifted itself off the surface of the table. It was all he could do to write his signature. What had started as an aggravation had now become a definite disability. Otherwise, he was in good health—perfect health, in fact. And he had no other complaints.

I asked him to write his signature for me.

As soon as he took his Cross pen out of his pocket, as soon as he grasped it, his fingers and thumb began to blanch from the force they were involuntarily exerting on the pen.

He started to write.

J

The fingers started to curl under.

o

s

e

The wrist began to flex.

p

h

By now, his last two fingers were digging into his palm. And his wrist was fully flexed, at a right angle to his forearm.

M

It took him almost a second to form the M.

a

r

His elbow started to lift off the table.

t

i

His fingertips and knuckles were almost pure white.

His elbow was six inches off the table.

n

He stopped—no Ph.D.

His elbow slowly lowered itself.

His wrist began to straighten out.

Color began to return to his fingers.

His fingers relaxed and became uncurled, and the pen fell from his loosened grasp.

"Once more," I said.

"Must I?" he asked.

"Yes, but with a difference," I replied. With that I reached into my pocket and pulled out a small, red object made out of a soft plastic. It was a cylinder with triangularly shaped outer walls. You can buy one at any school-supply store. They are made to help first graders hold their pencils. The pencil fits through the internal round cylinder, while the far larger triangular exterior is easier for the fingers to grasp. The entire object is about an inch and a half long.

I took Professor Martin's Cross pen and stuck it through the device. As I handed it back to him, I told him to write his signature.

He gingerly picked up the pen from the top of my desk, his fingers and thumb pressing against the pen holder.

J

The fingers began to curl, ever so slightly.

o

s

e

p

h

All his fingers were slightly bent.

M

Written in a flash.

a

r

t

i

n

There had been no flexing of the wrist, and his elbow was still resting on the table.

Without my asking, he kept on writing.

He wrote his signature several times and then began to write out Plato's *Death of Socrates*, which he had taught so often that he knew it by heart.

After five minutes, he had to stop, because the continuous mild cramp of his fingers was becoming uncomfortable.

"I'm cured," he said.

"No," I contradicted him. "But your symptoms are under reasonable control."

I tried to explain his disorder to him. He had what we call *dystonic writer's cramp*. A dystonia is any abnormal movement that causes a sustained abnormal posture. Most such dystonias are brought about by some sort of action. His came on while writing and resulted in a cramp, ergo dystonic writer's cramp.

"You have defined what I have, not explained it," Professor Martin protested.

He was correct. The problem was that I could not really explain his problem. All the classic movement disorders—Parkinson's disease, Huntington's chorea, Wilson's disease, dystonia—are due to abnormal function in parts of the brain that are referred to as the extrapyramidal system. The term *extrapyramidal system* is not old as far as medical concepts go. It was first used in 1912 by the English neurologist S. A. K. Wilson in his discussion of a "new" neurologic disorder associated with cirrhosis of the liver, which now bears his name (Wilson's disease—see "Still Smiling"). Wilson used this term to refer to those parts of the central nervous system that governed motor disorders but that were not a part of the two other principal motor systems, which were already well known: the pyramidal system and the cerebellar. The term has since come into general use, both clinically and anatomically, to refer to the third of the three principal motor systems in humans. Each of these three systems is conceptualized as a separate system entity made up of independent parts of the nervous system. Lesions within these systems result in distinctive disturbances of motor activity.

The pyramidal tract derives its name from the fact that the constituent fibers pass through a pyramid-shaped structure in the brain stem. Its fibers start in the cerebral cortex, principally from that area in the frontal lobe called the motor cortex. The fibers then descend through the brain stem and, after crossing to the other side of the nervous system, continue through the spinal cord and finally terminate on the lower motor neurons. These lower motor neurons in turn send messages to all the body's muscles. Injury to this tract produces paralysis of voluntary movement. As a result, the pyramidal system is believed to be concerned with the *initiation* of voluntary movements. The best-known example of a disease of this system is a classic cerebrovascular accident or stroke involving the pyramidal tract deep in one side of the brain, which causes paralysis of the opposite arm, leg, and side of the face.

The cerebellar system comprises the cerebellum and the pathways that bring information to it and relay its discharges. Lesions of this system result in tremors in movement, incoordination, and ataxia (imbalanced gait). The cerebellar system is believed to be concerned with the *coordination* of movements. The loss of coordination and imbalance that is seen in multiple sclerosis is due to cerebellar dysfunction, as are the analagous motor problems of simple drunkenness.

The extrapyramidal system is made up of a large collection of neurons (called nuclei) deep within the brain. These nuclei are all paired, there being one deep within each hemisphere. The major ones are the caudate nuclei, putamen, globus pallidus, substantia nigra, and subthalamic nuclei. The term *basal ganglia* is often used to refer to all these structures. Lesions of the extrapyramidal system often result in abnormal movements that are usually present at rest. Such lesions also lead to abnormalities of posture. This system is thought to be concerned primarily with the *maintenance of posture*, as opposed to the initiation or coordination of voluntary movement. It is responsible for the unconscious coordination of posture, which allows the body to carry out coordinated (cerebellar-controlled) conscious, purposeful movements initiated by the pyramidal tract.

"So why does my hand cramp up as soon as I pick up a pen?" he asked.

A good question.

I even had a pretty good answer. The ability of the various parts of the extrapyramidal system to maintain the appropriate postures is dependent upon a variety of sensory inputs into the brain. I used Parkinson's disease as an example. Patients with Parkinson's disease can walk through a room with little problem, but as they approach a doorway, they will start to bend forward more, and their posture will become more flexed, more stooped. Their strides become far shorter. Their feet do not lift as far off the ground. Rather, they shuffle, at times resulting in a sudden halt. Once they get through the doorway, the patients straighten up, their stride gets longer, and their feet no longer shuffle. This range of behaviors results from the effect of the visual input on the extrapyramidal system.

The same sort of phenomenon occurs in dystonia, which has been described best in a form of dystonia called *spasmodic torticollis*. Torticollis means torsion or turning of the neck. In torticollis, the abnormality consists of a dystonic movement that rotates the neck. Such patients often have no abnormal movements when lying in bed, but as soon as they begin to support their head, their neck starts into spasms, and their head is swung over to one side. The disability that such a dystonia causes is obvious. Professor Martin might be able to limit his writing, but what does one do if one's head turns to the right each time one stands up? These patients often use a trick or a gesture that they have learned independently: They touch their heads in a particular way, and the spasms decrease. It doesn't take much. The patient doesn't have to forcefully push on his or her head, but merely touches it. A finger to the cheek, a touch on the chin, a hand on the back of the head, and the neck muscles relax, and the head returns more toward its normal position.

Why?

The touch supplies information to the brain and in so doing changes the way the brain perceives the posture of the neck. That new perception corrects the abnormal message previously being sent out.

What happens, then, in writer's cramp?

At least two separate motor programs are involved in writing. One is the conscious initiation of finger movements needed to form the letters. This is a function of the pyramidal system. The other is the unconscious posturing of the fingers, hand, and arm to allow the pyramidal system to carry out the act of writing—an extrapyramidal function.

In dystonic writer's cramp, the act of writing itself is not affected. The pyramidal system functions normally. What *is* disrupted is the program for posturing, which is an abnormality of the extrapyramidal system, the same type of abnormality that occurs in spasmodic torticollis.

In torticollis, changing the overall input sent to the brain helps to control the symptoms. The same phenomenon holds true in dystonic writer's cramp: that, in effect, is what the little gadget did for Professor Martin. It changed the position of his fingers, and in so doing changed the message that his fingers sent to his brain. Sometimes that can influence the function of the extrapyramidal system enough to help control the dystonic symptoms.

That was what the pen holder did for Professor Martin. It changed the position of the fingers and thereby the message they sent to his brain and fortunately this new message was enough to change the function of his brain in the right direction.

The Cross pen had a similar effect, and it, too, had changed his symptoms. But not in the right direction—it had made his cramps worse.

"Is this a real disease?" Professor Martin now asked.

Another good question.

I'm not sure my answer was equally good. I discussed the entire concept of occupational dystonias—dystonias brought on by a particular occupation or activity, such as writing. Most of them, I am convinced, are not diseases.

I used my favorite example of a nondisease, the occupational dystonia of musicians. Some violinists, after hours and hours of playing get dystonic cramps in their left hands. Their left hands have a role similar to the role of the right hand in writing. As a result, the violinist develops an "abnormal" dystonic posture and can no longer execute the repeated finger movements needed to play the violin.

Is that a disease? Or merely excessive demand placed on the brain by playing the violin? Was the extrapyramidal system designed to play a violin for six or eight hours at a time?

Another example. In the 1984 Olympics, in the women's marathon, one of the contestants developed a dystonic cramp on one side of her body as she neared the finish line.

Marathon runner's dystonia, an occupational dystonia of marathon runners. Is that a disease? Or an overstressed brain.

I tend to think that such instances represent the limited ability of normal brains to continue to process information correctly under conditions of excessive demand. I do not consider such disorders as diseases per se, for a disease implies abnormality. Writer's cramp is part of the same process.

David Marsden, of the Neurologic Institute in London, and one of the world's leading authorities on the physiology of movement disorders, I know, disagrees. He regards all forms of dystonia as abnormal and hence as disease. So do others. That's what keeps our scientific meetings so interesting.

We were done with our visit, and Professor Martin got up to leave.

"That'll be twenty-five cents," I said.

"For the consultation?"

"No, for the holder. I have to get another."

"Can't you charge your next patient for that one?"

"It's not for a patient," I said. "It's for me. I have a dystonic writer's cramp."

"Is that why you believe it's not a disease?"

"No comment," I replied.

=11=

The Great American Opera

Listen, bud, take my advice. Never hate a song that has sold a half-million copies.
—Irving Berlin, said to Cole Porter

Opera in English is, in the main, just about as sensible as baseball in Italian.
—H. L. Mencken

Everyone's famous for fifteen minutes.
—Andy Warhol

One of the greatest disappointments during my four years of medical school was that I was never taught precisely what a nervous breakdown is. None of my professors ever mentioned the term, nor did my textbooks. Nor did any of the articles I read in the scientific journals. What made this one disappointment more distressing than the usual day-to-day frustrations of medical school was the obvious fact that everyone I knew who wasn't a medical student seemed to understand the term quite clearly.

My mother certainly did. Of course, she was a nurse.

So did my wife. Of course, she was married to a medical student.

Even my old college roommate did—and he was in law school and didn't know any doctors or medical students except me.

They had all known about nervous breakdowns for years. They had acquaintances who had nervous breakdowns. They had read about other people who had suffered from them. We have all read these stories, about people both famous and not so famous, and drawn our own conclusions.

It's just that I needed to know exactly what a nervous breakdown was in medical terms.

Is a nervous breakdown neurologic? Is it psychiatric? What happens in the brain? What happens to the patient? Is it an acute attack of schizophrenia? Or mania? Or depression? Or hysteria?

Everyone else understood: It's a nervous breakdown, a psychiatric problem, not a neurologic disease. And most patients got better.

In the years since medical school, I have learned more about nervous breakdowns, not from textbooks or scientific articles, but by reading the histories of individuals who suffered from them. One of these individuals has come to be recognized as among America's most successful composers, a writer of popular songs who yearned to write the Great American Opera.

I am not referring to George Gershwin—America's greatest composer, who went from Tin Pan Alley to Carnegie Hall and later on to *Porgy and Bess*—but to Scott Joplin. Joplin, like Gershwin, was a remarkably successful composer of "pop" songs who wanted to create something more significant. Joplin wanted to succeed in the world of serious music. He wanted to compose the first great American opera.

Only he did it twenty years before Gershwin.

Joplin was born in Texarkana, Arkansas, in 1868, just after the Civil War. Joplin was black; his parents had both been slaves. Joplin initially studied piano in Arkansas and by the mid-1880s was traveling and performing widely in the Midwest. In 1893, he performed at the Columbian Exposition in Chicago.

In 1895, he began studying music at the George R. Smith College for Negroes, hoping for a career as a concert pianist and classical composer. His first published songs quickly brought him fame, and in 1900, he moved to St. Louis to work with the music publisher John Stark.

Joplin published his first extended work, a ballet suite using all the rhythmic devices of ragtime, with his own choreographic directions, in 1902. His first opera, *A Guest of Honor* (1903), was lost by the copyright office. After moving to New York City in 1907, Joplin wrote an instruction book, *The School of Ragtime,* outlining his complex bass patterns, sporadic syncopation, stop-time breaks, and harmonic ideas, which were already being widely imitated. Many American pop composers used these techniques, including Irving Berlin ("Alexander's Ragtime Band"), Gershwin, and others. Twenty years later, classical composers followed suit.

Joplin's contract with Stark ended in 1909, and though he made some piano rolls in his final years, most of his efforts during this period involved *Treemonisha,* a work that synthesized all his musical ideas into a conventional three-act opera. Joplin wrote the libretto, concerning a mythical black leader, and choreographed it as well. *Treemonisha* had only one semipublic performance during Joplin's lifetime; he became obsessed by his efforts to succeed with it, and suffered a nervous breakdown in 1911. He never recovered from it and was finally institutionalized in 1916.

Joplin had far more than a run-of-the-mill nervous breakdown, however. In fact, he did not have a psychiatric problem at all, but a progressive neurologic disease that first affected his sanity and ultimately killed him. His disease carries the long name general paresis of the insane (GPI for short). In the years before penicillin was discovered, this was the commonest way that syphilis caused significant neurologic disorders. GPI was so common that at the turn of the century, it was the most frequent cause—more common than either schizophrenia or Alzheimer's disease—of severe mental illness requiring institutionalization in a psychiatric facility.

GPI was once a common form of nervous breakdown. The French writer Guy du Maupassant and the German poet Heinrich Heine died from it, as did tens of thousands of others, most of whom were not famous at all. GPI was such an urgent health problem that the Nobel Prize in medicine (the first ever awarded to a psychiatrist) was given to the Viennese psychiatrist who devised the first successful form of treatment for it. His name became a household word, and his face even appeared on an Austrian banknote.

His name? Not Sigmund Freud, but Wagner von Jauregg. His name is no longer a household word, even in his native Vienna, and his contribution to medicine is now an all but forgotten part of the history of medicine. His contribution: fever therapy for general paresis of the insane. He successfully treated syphilis of the brain by causing the patients to run high-grade fevers for several days.

General paresis of the insane was a progressive, uniformly fatal mental illness that developed in patients five to twenty years after their original syphilitic infection. General paretics are exceedingly rare in mental hospitals today, but that was not always the case. In a world that is just beginning to face the problems brought on by an epidemic of a venereal disease that also commonly involves the brain (AIDS), the history of syphilis, which, like AIDS, began as an acute epidemic, is more than just a historical curiosity.

Although general paresis was not recognized as a specific disease until the eighteen twenties, syphilis is generally accepted to have become a major health problem in Europe in the sixteenth century. Syphilis seems to have first appeared in Europe shortly after the return of Christopher Columbus and his crew from their first trip to the New World. Whether the dissemination was due to the activities of the former or the latter remains open to conjecture, but it is clear that the first cases appeared in Spain shortly after Columbus and his ships returned there.

The New World origin of syphilis, while accepted by almost all contemporary authorities, later came under attack by some medical historians. The records of the spread of the disease and the observations of late fifteenth- and sixteenth-century physicians and historians make an overwhelming case for the so-called Haitian hypothesis. This theory suggests that Columbus's crew consorted with and "knew" native women in Haiti, contracted the disease there, and brought it back with them to Spain, from where it was disseminated throughout Europe.

A single military campaign played a major role in spreading this devastating new disease. In fall 1494, Charles VIII, the King of France, invaded Italy in pursuit of his claim to the throne of the Kingdom of Naples. Italy was then composed of numerous city states and petty kingdoms whose strength had been sapped by constant internecine rivalry. King Charles met no effective resistance during his initial advance into Italy, and his army easily marched down the peninsula all the way to Naples. Charles's forces were composed of mercenaries from many parts of Western Europe, including French, German, Swiss, English, Hungarian, Polish, Italian, and, of course, Spanish contingents. This 30,000-man army was accompanied by a thousand or more "camp followers"—merely a euphemism for prostitutes. The march to Naples was more a parade of debauchery than a serious military campaign. In late 1494, Charles began his siege of Naples. In army camps at that time, sexual diversions were an expected and welcome change of pace. The women often moved freely from one side to the other, and Spanish mercenaries were present in both Charles's army and among the defenders of Naples. Under these circumstances, the spread of a new venereal disease is easy to comprehend. Gabriel Fallopius, the great anatomist who gave his name to the fallopian tubes, described how the defenders of Naples "finally with violence drove their harlots and women out of the citadel, and especially the most beautiful ones, whom they knew to be suffering from the infectious disease, on the pretext that the food had come to an end. And the French, gripped by compassion and bewitched by their beauty, took them in." By spring 1495, this new disease accomplished something the Italians could not: Charles's army had been devastated, and Charles was forced to retreat. The withdrawal back up the Italian peninsula presented a great contrast with the almost triumphant advance of the previous fall. Charles's army disintegrated into undisciplined lawless bands, which fled northward and scattered into France, Switzerland, Germany, and their other homelands, bringing their new disease with them. Step by step, syphilis appeared in France, Germany, Switzerland in 1495 and in Holland and Greece in 1496. It spread to England and Scotland in 1497 and to Hungary and Russia in 1499. In recognition of the source of the disaster, the new affliction was first called the Neapolitan disease, but later became known as the French disease. Charles VIII died from it in 1498 at the age of only twenty-eight.

Syphilis was originally described as an illness that was usually of venereal origin. In contrast to all other such maladies, it almost always developed into much more than a genital infection, causing severe rashes and generalized symptoms often resulting in death. Up to that time, physicians had been aware only of purely local genital afflictions. It is striking that in all medieval and ancient sources, there is not one definite reference to a venereal/genital disease involving more widespread signs and symptoms. This peculiar feature of syphilis was recognized by contemporaries as definite evidence that syphilis was a new entity.

The severity of syphilis during its initial epidemic phase also provides good evidence of the newness of this disease in Europe. It is virtually an axiom in the history of disease that when an infectious illness first appears among a people, it appears with greater severity in terms of both morbidity and mortality than it ordinarily causes in people already exposed and adapted to the disease. This tendency has been recorded many times and in many places for such diseases as measles, scarlet fever, smallpox, and even in modern epidemics of syphilis among isolated peoples. It may in part be the case today for AIDS.

In contrast with the almost trivial character of the early manifestations of syphilis when it occurs today, all evidence points to its severe character during its first epidemic at the end of the fifteenth century. Most cases presented with a severe, acute disorder with high fever, intense headache and bone and joint pains, early skin rashes so severe that they stimulated smallpox, great prostration, and frequently an early death. The epidemic thus had all the characteristics of a virulent plague. Given the morals of the time, the "syphilization" of much of Europe occurred rapidly, and many contemporaries noticed that the severity of the symptoms of early syphilis quickly diminished. Within fifty years, the disease assumed the character with which the world has since been familiar.

Syphilis as a disease widespread in Western Europe dates back to the 1490s, but GPI was not identified until some 300 years later. How can we explain this late date for the first recognition of syphilis of the brain? The delay of 300 years between the recognition of acute syphilis and that of GPI is the result of many factors. First, there was an increased interest in insanity in the early nineteenth century. This interest was associated historically with the teachings of Esquirol (1772–1840), who emphasized the value of careful observation and detailed case recording and stressed the need to break down the old trinity of madness (mania, melancholia, dementia) into discrete, well-defined illnesses. Second, the establishment of mental hospitals during that era made it possible for patients with severe psychiatric illnesses to be observed over long periods of time. Finally, the rise of the field of pathology encouraged careful postmortem examinations of the brain. GPI itself is associated with characteristic changes within the brain. Its distinct clinical features—seizures, progressive paralysis, and severe dementia—could all be traced to identifiable pathological lesions. This brought psychiatry to the same level as other branches of medicine, in which signs and symptoms were finally being associated with specific structural pathology. Syphilis even became the model psychiatric disease.

All these factors may be part of the explanation why syphilis of the brain was not recognized for 300 years. But it may be equally true that GPI was virtually absent during that period. How can this absence of a natural phase of syphilis be explained? Perhaps nature anticipated von Jauregg and used the same method he used to treat GPI—the induction of recurrent high fevers to prevent the occurrence of the disease.

Numerous infectious illnesses associated with high fevers were widespread in the Europe of fifteenth, sixteenth, seventeenth, eighteenth, and even nineteenth centuries. These included malaria, smallpox, relapsing fever, typhus, and others. As early as 1539, one medical authority suggested that a high fever, such as that caused by malaria, might arrest syphilis. At one time, malaria was a common disease in Europe. Pandemics of malaria recurred for centuries after the introduction of syphilis, the last appearing between 1855 and 1873. It is reasonable to assume that better methods of treatment shortened the duration of malaria in many patients in the later pandemics and thus reduced the prophylactic effect of fever associated with it. The prophylactic benefit of malaria can best be appreciated by looking outside Europe, where there is fairly convincing evidence that the presence of malaria in various areas has provided the population of those regions with reasonable protection against the late neurologic complications of syphilis.

But malaria was not the only prophylactic fever, and probably has not been the most important source of prevention. Smallpox is also likely to have played a major role, and it was smallpox that helped stimulate von Jauregg's imagination.

Smallpox is characterized by two distinct bouts of fever. The first one consists of temperatures up to 41–42 degrees centigrade for three or four days during the prodromal stage. Then, if the case is uncomplicated, a second episode of milder fever for nine or ten days occurs during the stage of eruption. Because of the nature of the fever it causes, smallpox would provide excellent protection against general paresis. But was smallpox common enough in Europe before the end of the eighteenth century and the widespread use of vaccination to have afforded protection from GPI? It certainly was. Smallpox is reported to have killed 45 million of Europe's 165 million inhabitants in the eighteenth century. Most Europeans contracted the disease. With the advent of large-scale vaccination against smallpox, the rate of the disease finally declined, and as it did, more and more general paresis began to appear.

This correlation was convincingly documented in 1926, the year before Julius Wagner von Jauregg won the Nobel Prize, by a Ukrainian psychiatrist, L. Daraszkiewicz, who reported that during fifteen years of psychiatry in the Ukraine, he had not seen a single patient with GPI who had scars from smallpox. During this same period, he saw these scars in numerous patients who were suffering from other mental diseases. Moreover, he had never seen a patient with GPI who did not have a scar from a smallpox vaccination. His conclusions on the basis of these observations were twofold. First, he believed that unvaccinated individuals could hardly avoid contracting smallpox and that smallpox gave them "absolute" protection against GPI. Second, he believed that syphilis could not lead to general paresis unless the victim had been "tainted" with cowpox, that is, vaccinated against smallpox. Daraszkiewicz drew attention to the fact that there was practically no general paresis in Europe from 1500 to 1800, although syphilis was common, and that the same was still true in areas that were not yet touched by modern European civilization and its associated vaccinations. Daraszkiewicz was widely attacked for his views, and although his contention that vaccination made syphilis more likely to cause GPI remains unproved, the protective role of smallpox seems clear.

Relapsing fevers are a group of infectious diseases that may have played a similar role. In Europe, at that time relapsing fever was usually transmitted by lice. Epidemics occurred in various parts of Europe in the eighteenth century and in Russia and Ireland in the nineteenth century.

Tick-borne typhus, another epidemic disease, most likely played an even greater part in preventing GPI, but at a much greater cost. Typhus is characterized by prolonged high fever, sometimes lasting for as long as ten days. This fever has a strongly deleterious effect on Treponema pallidum, the bacterium that causes syphilis. Young people seldom die of the disease, but the mortality rate rises with age to over 60 percent. The disease is especially prevalent during times of war, and caused great havoc in Europe in the seventeenth and eighteenth centuries. A widespread epidemic developed in the wake of Napoleon's retreat from Moscow in 1812 and spread over most of Europe.

It was not until the early nineteenth century that GPI was recognized as a specific disease, and within fifty years, it had become relatively common. In the meantime, great advances had been made in the diagnosis of syphilis, but treatment lagged far behind. It was only in 1910 that Paul Ehrlich (1854–1915) introduced "606" (salvarsan) a "salvation" arsenical that he found in his 606th experiment. It was unique in that it was the first medicine that destroyed the causative spirochete within the patient's body. Despite its efficiency in the early stages of syphilis, salvarsan was of little, if any, value in treating GPI.

Julius Wagner von Jauregg (1857–1940) must be given full credit for developing the first truly effective form of therapy of central nervous system syphilis. He was born in Wels, Austria. His father was a state official there and was named only Wagner until he was knighted and added the von Jauregg. Wagner von Jauregg studied medicine at the University of Vienna, receiving his degree in 1880. After graduation, he continued to work in the Institute of Pathology until 1883, when he accepted a position in a psychiatric clinic, but apparently only after he had failed to obtain a similar position in internal medicine. While working at the clinic, he discovered that several patients with mental symptoms improved after suffering an acute attack of typhoid fever. In 1887, he wrote an article suggesting that patients who suffered from psychoses should be treated by infecting them with febrile disease, such as malaria or erysipelas. He himself failed to induce erysipelas in some of his patients by injecting a culture of streptococci. After Robert Koch discovered tuberculin, von Jauregg used it to produce fever, but abandoned it as too dangerous.

Wagner von Jauregg moved to Graz in 1889 to become head of the department of psychiatry of the university. In 1892, he returned to Vienna, as chief of the Psychiatric Clinic of the Allgemeine Krankenhaus. In 1902, he succeeded Richard von Krafft-Ebing as professor of neurology and psychiatry at the University of Vienna. Despite increasing responsibilities and broadening interests, von Jauregg never lost sight of the possibility of treating psychosis with fever. Two phyicians in the Austrian Army J. Mattauchek and A. Pilcz reported on their long-term follow-up of over 4,000 officers in the Imperial Austrian Army who developed syphilis. They noted that about 5 percent eventually developed GPI. Not a single instance of GPI developed among the 241 officers who subsequently contracted an acute infectious disease, such as malaria, pneumonia, or typhoid fever within a few years of contracting syphilis. Without any such prophylactic event, the expected number of cases of GPI in these 241 officers would have been about a dozen.

Wagner von Jauregg was impressed by these data and by the observation that general paresis did not occur in countries where malaria was endemic. Finally, as World War I waned, he put his general theory into specific practice. In that year, he inoculated "benign tertian" malaria organisms into patients with GPI. This procedure was not submitted to any Committee on Human Investigation, nor were any informed consents obtained, but it worked. Of the nine patients von Jauregg treated, six definitely benefited, and three of them were still working four years later. For his discovery of the therapeutic value of malaria inoculation in the treatment of general paresis of the insane, Wagner von Jauregg was awarded the Nobel Prize for physiology and medicine in 1927. He was the first, and to date the only, psychiatrist to receive this honor.

Von Jauregg's discovery came far too late to help Scott Joplin. When Joplin became ill, there was no effective treatment that could arrest the progress of GPI. Joplin became another victim of GPI.

People still get nervous breakdowns today, and I'm still not sure what they have. It is, however, most unlikely that they are suffering from GPI. The disease is rarely seen today and syphilis itself has been in part displaced by a new venereal epidemic, AIDS. But the displacement has not been complete. The only case of GPI I have seen in the past five years occurred in a patient with AIDS. His immune abnormalities undoubtedly made it far easier for the bacteria that cause GPI to enter his brain.

That fatal epidemic diseases can be caused by illicit sexual intercourse has been recognized for almost five hundred years. Neither the inherent threat to health nor the associated moral preaching seems to have done much to change human behavior. Clearly, more effective forms of prevention must be found. Von Jauregg found one for GPI. Let us hope that one is found for AIDS far more quickly.

Author's Note

There are so many sources on the history of syphilis that any choice of references must reflect the prejudices of the selector. Alfred Crosby's "The Early History of Syphilis" (*American Anthropologist* 71 [1969]: 218-27) gives a balanced appraisal of the sources. Somewhat greater documentation can be found in William A. Pussey's *The History of the Epidemiology of Syphilis* (Springfield Ill.: Charles C Thomas, 1933), which remains my favorite. The only complete discussion of the inverse relationship between GPI and other infectious diseases is Bernard Jacobowsky's "General Paresis and Civilization" (*Acta Psychiatrica Scandinavica* 41 [1965]: 267-73.)

12

The Bobbsey Twins Take Neurology

Niels Bohr, the brilliant twentieth-century atomic physicist, had a horseshoe nailed to the wall of his house. Other scientists were scandalized by this behavior; they could not believe that Bohr accepted such superstitions. He always replied that he didn't. "But," he would add, "I've been told they work even if you don't believe in them."

Their classmates in medical school always called them "the twins." I'm told that at first they were referred to as "the Bobbsey Twins," and that that had originally been a term of derision. They were actually husband and wife and had been married since the summer before medical school. They were both from downstate Illinois, somewhere around Cairo, and had grown up together, gone to the same high school, been childhood sweethearts, gone to the same college, married, and were now classmates in medical school. Neither Martin nor Mary Rickert had hayseed in his or her hair—at least not that I ever noticed—but their speech was peppered with such phrases as "gosh," "gee whiz," and "golly," with an occasional "so's your old man." They were right out of *The Music Man*.

They were too sweet and too endearing for the derision to last. The gee whizes persisted, but "the Bobbsey Twins" gave way to "the Twins." The latter implied no derision; it merely described them to a "T." They were virtually twins. They did everything together; they went everywhere together. They had the same mannerisms. Their clothes always seemed to match.

I first got to know them when I lectured to their class on neuropharmacology during their second year in medical school. Pharmacology is the study of medications and how they act in treating various diseases. Neuropharmacology is that segment of pharmacology that deals with the treatment of neurologic diseases. I gave a course of ten lectures, a series that didn't cover all neurology but did manage to include a survey of all neuropharmacology, for there are many neurologic diseases for which there are no specific treatments. Disorders like amyotrophic lateral sclerosis (also called Lou Gehrig's disease), cerebral hemorrhage, and Frederick's (hereditary) ataxia have no treatment, and were never mentioned in my lectures. Other diseases, such as multiple sclerosis, are treated with drugs that are primarily used to treat nonneurologic disorders and were discussed elsewhere in the pharmacology curriculum. As a result, I discussed multiple sclerosis only in passing. That did not concern me, since the effectiveness of much of what we do in treating the disease is far from proved. My lectures focused instead on those diseases with specfific therapeutics: epilepsy, Parkinson's disease, and migraine headache, to name a few of the more prominent disorders.

Both the twins loved my classes. It was a love that came as a surprise to both of them. During my first lecture, they sat toward the back of the hall, near the aisle, for easy exit in case things got dull. That practice is common in medical schools today. Attendance at lectures is no longer compulsory, and students are given printed copies of all lectures. The students tend to show up for a teacher's first lecture. If it's boring, they often disappear to return only when a new lecturer appears. Bill Veeck had observed the same phenomenon when he owned the St. Louis Browns (of sainted memory): "No one came to opening day, and after that the attendance dwindled rapidly."

The twins showed up at all ten lectures. By the third one, they were sitting in the middle of the second row. By the fifth, they were coming down afterwards to ask me questions—questions still peppered with "goshes" and "gees," but good questions, nonetheless.

Their interest in neurology/neuropharmacology did not end when that course was over—far from it. The lectures had kindled their interest and enthusiasm, and neurology became one more shared part of their lives. Over the next several months, they stopped by my office practically every week to ask questions, to borrow books, to clarify concepts. Always together. Always reading the same chapters and asking the same questions.

Toward early spring, they asked for jobs. In fact, they asked for two identical jobs doing research in my laboratory over the summer. At that time, I had funds for only one summer research fellow. Ordinarily, I took one student and assigned him or her to a single specific project. That way, I had sufficient time to devote to the student to make that summer job a learning experience. And I also had limited space in my lab. Too many students cluttered the place up and put far too much strain on my technicians, who also had to tutor them. I'd tried two students the previous year, and it had been a technical disaster. My staff made me promise—only one student this summer.

Mary and Martin both wanted jobs. That meant two salaries, two projects, two spaces in my laboratory. Twice as much of my time to supervise them. And twice as much of my technicians' time, with the inevitable chaos in the lab.

I couldn't do it. One was the limit. But which one? I couldn't tell them apart. Which would fit in better? Which was more interested? Which was more likely to profit from the experience? To become a neurologist?

The latter was a valid question. I used those summer fellowships as proving grounds for future residents. But which one would be a better resident? I had no idea. They were as alike as twins, identical twins of opposite sexes. Biologically impossible, but this wasn't biology, this was medical school. And how could I separate "the Twins?" Castor without Pollux. I couldn't, and I suspected they wouldn't let me.

When I raised the practical problems to them, they told me they were willing to settle for one project, sharing time with me and the one salary. That solved only part of the difficulty: the matter of the laboratory remained. I had made a solemn promise to my technicians.

I gave in. They would work together on a single project, which would require two work places in the lab. And, I insisted, two salaries. I would find the extra money somewhere. I had no idea where my technicians would find space for them or the time to supervise them. It would be a disaster again.

Except it wasn't. The technicians loved them, their genuine enthusiasm for science, and their infectious innocence. And the twins loved their summer. By the fall, I knew it had been a success. Both Martin and Mary had decided to become neurologists.

That November, they began their clerkship in neurology. Four solid weeks of seeing patients with neurologic disorders. That experience did nothing to dampen their enthusiasm, and, in fact, sharpened their focus. They both decided that they wanted to take their residencies with us.

I was thrilled: they would both be great residents. The patients loved them, and they were already learning to be excellent doctors. They would be a pleasure to have around for three years. Golly gee!

I was finishing rounds on a Monday about two weeks after the twins completed their clerkships when Mary paged me. She wanted to talk to me about something personal. It was almost noon, and since I was free until one or so I told her to meet me at my office.

Mary arrived first and was waiting for me, seated in a chair in my office. Her eyes were reddened; she had obviously been crying. Her face was pale. Her legs were crossed, but her top leg kept kicking up and down, betraying her obvious agitation.

"What's wrong?" I asked.

"I can't see out of my right eye," she said in a single burst, and then began crying.

"Did you see an ophthalmologist?" I asked.

She nodded, biting her upper lip in an attempt to combat the tears.

"What did he see?"

"Nothing," she whispered.

"Damn," I said without thinking.

"Yes," she said. "Damn."

I had never previously heard her say anything remotely that strong.

I waited until she was ready to talk and then listened as she told me what had happened. It had started when she had gotten up the previous Saturday morning. Things didn't look right to her; they seemed blurry, fuzzy. She knew enough neurology to know what to do next. She closed her right eye, and everything looked fine—sharp and clear. Then she closed her left eye. All she could see were the objects on the periphery. Straight ahead, everything was black, a great black hole in front of her right eye.

Except it wasn't really in front of her eye. As a medical student, she'd studied the anatomy of the brain and neurology and knew that the hole was actually behind her eye.

The pathway that conveys vision from the eyes to the brain is complex, but it is that very complexity that makes it easy to define the precise location of a visual problem, once you know the rules. And Mary knew the rules.

Mary's visual disorder was limited to her right eye. Therefore, her problem had to be either in her right eye itself or in the nerve directly behind her right eye—the right optic nerve.

Because the ophthalmologist had looked into her eye and had seen nothing that was abnormal, the difficulty had to be in her optic nerve, at a point directly behind the eye. This part of the nerve is called retrobulbar, meaning behind the bulb (of the eye). And from her history and age and the nature of her complaint, there could only be one cause: retrobulbar neuritis, inflammation of the retrobulbular optic nerve.

She already knew all that, and more. She also knew that retrobulbar neuritis is often a precursor of multiple sclerosis, one of the most mysterious and frightening of all neurologic disorders.

Mary's visit took place in 1972, a time when every night the television featured ads proclaiming MS the "crippler of young adults." Mary Rickert had seen patients in the hospital with severe MS, and knew a little about it. A little knowledge is a dangerous thing.

I tried to reassure her even before I examined her. She needed it; I needed it. I went through my litany of facts.

Only one-third of patients with retrobulbar neuritis develop MS. Of course, it was not the two-thirds who didn't have the disease that the TV ads talked about. It was also not those two-thirds whom she had seen in the hospital during her neurology clerkship. It was the other one-third, especially that subgroup who had the severest forms of the disease with the worst prognosis.

Even if she developed MS, I told her, it could take ten or twenty years for her first real attack. I reassured her that many patients had MS without being crippled by it. Most went on that way for many years, and a good number forever.

Everything I said was true, true and irrelevant.

She told me a few more facts. Six months earlier, while she and Martin were home on vacation, her right leg and foot had felt funny for about two weeks. For several days, her foot didn't do what she wanted. By the time they returned to Chicago, she was virtually back to normal and getting better every day.

She never saw a doctor and never even told Martin about it.

She knew her diagnosis. She had MS. She had already had an attack, six months before she developed retrobulbar neuritis.

Today we have a number of sophisticated tests to confirm a diagnosis of MS. Note the verb—*confirm*. The diagnosis itself is based on clinical criteria. To make a diagnosis of MS, the doctor must know that the patient has a history of multiple (two or more) episodes of neurologic problems separated by time (six months for Mary) and space. The latter means that the lesions within the brain and spinal cord that are producing a patient's symptoms must be in separate locations. Mary's were. The lesion behind her right eye was, neurologically speaking, miles away from the one that had caused her leg and foot to feel funny.

Two episodes, separated in time and space.

She had MS.

The term MS was originally invented to describe the a condition that involved many areas of scarring or sclerosis in the nervous system. MS is now classified as a demyelinating disease. Myelin is the fatty membranous material that covers the nerve fibers and acts as insulation for them. MS, whatever it is—and we still don't know precisely its nature—attacks the myelin and affects the nerves within, which now no longer carry their messages correctly. When the myelin of the optic nerve is the site of the attack, retrobulbar neuritis develops, and vision in that eye deteriorates. Attacks come and go; we don't know why they do so. If the amount of myelin involved is limited, then an attack can clear without leaving any symptoms or changes in the neurologic exam. If the episode is more severe, however, permanent injury can be done, and areas of scarring are formed—patches of sclerosis. MS.

Today we can see those patches on NMR scans. In 1972, we had no NMRs, or CAT scans, either.

We did, however, have neurologic exams, and so I examined Mary.

Mary's first attack had not left her unscathed. The reflexes in her right leg were abnormally increased.

I had all I needed.

Mary had had two attacks separated in time and space.

We both knew she had MS, and while there were still a few tests we had to do, they would not change the facts.

"Can I do them as an outpatient?" she requested.

She could, even the spinal tap, which I did that afternoon in my office. It wasn't until the tap was completed that I became concerned by the fact that Martin, her nonbiological twin, had not made an appearance. I had noted that she had come to my office alone that morning but had assumed that Martin had some medical obligation he could not avoid, such as teaching rounds on a clinical service or scrubbing in on a surgical procedure. There were dozens of such things. When he didn't accompany her for the tap, I became curious. Perhaps he was on one of the killer clerkships, and it was impossible for him to steal away for even ten minutes. After the tap, Mary stayed in the office flat on her back for the requisite three hours until it was time for her to go home. It was now six o'clock, and still no Martin.

I finally asked her what clerkship Martin was on.

"Radiology," she said. "We both are."

No night call. The radiologists went home before four. Getting away for half an hour during the day was standard operating procedure. I didn't ask for any more details. I didn't have to.

The results of her spinal tap showed nothing. Today's tests would probably have shown an abnormality. We now look for what are called "oligoclonal bands"—abnormal antibodies within the spinal fluid. The process of MS seems to be dependent upon the production of these bands, which attack the myelin, causing demyelination. Why they are there remains a mystery, as does why they suddenly attack the myelin.

All recent research in therapy has focused on attempts to control the production of such antibodies, yet even in that area, we are uncertain if such approaches will be successful in controlling MS. All we had in 1972, however, were steroids.

I offered Mary a course of steroids. She wanted to talk to Martin first. She came back to see me the next day, agreeing to the treatment. I put her on steroids, and in two weeks her vision was back to normal.

Had the improvement been due to the steroids? Or the natural course of her disease? It was probably a combination of the two, and as to which was more significant, your guess is as good as mine.

If it was the natural course of her disease, however, then her disease was treating her well. That soon changed.

Mary had three serious attacks or exacerbations over the next two years. All three involved the brain stem; all three were equally dramatic and frightening. And all three had the same symptoms: slurred speech, drunken gait (ataxia), and inability to control her urine.

The first exacerbation took three months to clear up, the second and third even longer.

But all three did clear up, and quite well. Her speech went back to normal, as did her walking, as long as she wore flat-heel shoes. And she could control her urine.

Mary spent so much time in and out of the hospital that she finished medical school six months behind her class. She would be a year behind in starting her internship and her residency.

Martin hadn't waited for her, but had begun his internship right on time.

As soon as he had learned of her diagnosis, their relationship changed. When her first major attack struck, he moved out. They were divorced before her second one hit her. Martin graduated and took a neurology residency someplace else, but I never bothered to ask where. He never officially applied to our program, and it's just as well, for I wouldn't have taken him. That would have been an insult to one of my favorite patients. He had severed the tie that had connected the Bobbsey twins, and it was best if each went his own way. Last I heard he was on his second or third wife.

Mary didn't go into neurology, but stayed in Chicago and became a dermatologist. She felt that even if she had trouble walking, she could function well in that profession.

She got married in 1976 and now has one child. In 1980, she asked my advice about getting pregnant. We discussed the effect of pregnancy on MS. I told her that patients have a somewhat decreased chance of an attack during the nine months of pregnancy and a somewhat greater chance during the next three months, but overall the year is not much more hazardous than any other year for most. But for Mary, the more relevant issue was whether she'd be able to raise a child.

I could not give her an answer. She'd had no attacks in six years, which we both felt was a good sign, and she had no real disability—another good sign.

Her little girl is now seven. When her daughter was six years old, Mary had another attack, one that wasn't so kind. She now drags her left leg when she walks.

But if you ask her how she's doing, she replies, 'Gosh, life's been great.'' She has her career and her family, and she's enjoying both each day of her life.

She comes to see me once every three months and never misses a visit. I never ask her about symptoms; if she has any, she tells me. I only examine her if she is having new symptoms. This has happened only once in the past decade.

We talk as old friends.

It took several years for her to feel comfortable enough to tell me this story: When she had her first major attack and Martin Rickert of unsainted memory fled from the scene, one of her classmates visited her in the hospital and gave her a present—a piece of blue ribbon. It had come from Rachel's Tomb, outside Jerusalem. According to Jewish folklore, if a ribbon is wrapped around Rachel's Tomb and a certain prayer is said, pieces of that blue ribbon will preserve the health of the owner. Since then, Mary has kept that ribbon with her. She put it into a locket and still wears it around her neck.

''But you're not Jewish,'' I protested.

''The ribbon doesn't know that.''

''You don't believe in it, do you?'' I asked.

She didn't answer, so I told her about Niels Bohr and his horseshoe, which I thought was a funny story.

She laughed, but only to be polite. I never brought up the subject of the blue ribbon again. However, the last time I visited Israel, I went to Rachel's Tomb and acquired some pieces of blue ribbon. Every once in a while, when I have a young, distraught patient with MS, I tell him or her the story, and if the response is right, I give the patient a piece of ribbon. Why not? It can't hurt. After all, Niels Bohr did win the Nobel Prize in physics.

Author's Note

I heard Bill Veeck's reminiscence about the paid attendance in St. Louis on a radio interview. I do not know whether it was ever published. It has become part of the folklore of baseball.

13

He Died Old

The key to longevity is to keep breathing.
—Sophie Tucker

Mithradates, he died old.
—A. E. Housman, *A Shropshire Lad*

I glanced down at the patient information sheet, which was on the top of his chart, as he walked into my office. Aside from his name, John Brohamer, and his age, seventy-seven, the sheet contained no other information that was of any use to me in my role as a diagnostician. I had not seen him previously. Whenever a patient comes to me for the first time, for an "initial neurologic evaluation," that patient has sought me out to obtain my opinion about either his or her diagnosis or about the proper management of his or her known neurologic condition. In both instances, my initial responsibility is to make the correct diagnosis, if possible. Much of what I have to do to accomplish that depends upon direct observation, so by habit, I begin to make my observations even before I say hello to the patient.

Mr. Brohamer walked vigorously into my office, swinging his arms freely and moving with long confident strides, lifting both feet well off the ground. Already I knew that his gait showed no evidence of significant neurologic disorder—no hemiplegia from a stroke, no parkinsonism, no marked weakness of his legs from nerve or muscle disease. Were it not for the deep furrows and crags that cut across his face, I would have guessed his age as somewhere around sixty or sixty-five. Or as we say in the trade: He appeared to be at least a dozen years younger than his stated age.

I introduced myself and asked, "What seems to be the problem, Mr. Brohamer?"

"I'm getting old," he began, and then stopped.

I waited, but he said nothing more. "True," I replied. "We are all getting older, but what seems to be the problem?" I was not in any way trying to trivialize the difficulties associated with normal aging, but patients come to neurologists because of some symptom or group of symptoms that they or someone else perceive as not being part of the normal life cycle.

"But that is the problem," he protested. "I am getting old and as I get old, each system of my body, each and every organ, is itself getting old and I want to do whatever I can to alter that process. I have already seen a cardiologist and an endocrinologist, and now I am seeing a neurologist. The brain is, of course, one of the organs I am most concerned about preserving."

"Of course," I nodded. He had gone to see a cardiologist first. That was reasonable, given the high incidence of heart disease in the aging population in the United States. Then an endocrinologist. That did not seem quite as logical, but I didn't ask any questions about that.

"I chose you because you specialize in the neurological diseases of . . . ," he hesitated, groping for the right phrase, ". . . the aging population and have written about preventing the progression of some of those diseases."

He was right on both counts.

"What can you do to help me?"

It was not a question that healthy individuals asked of me, but it was not an entirely novel question, either. It represented one of man's perennial concerns. John Brohamer was not Ponce de León seeking a fountain of youth, nor was he necessarily trying to prolong his life. He simply wanted to keep his body from aging as long as he could.

But what is aging?

Why does the body age?

Why were so many of his individual organs aging?

In general terms, I cannot give any answers to these questions. In relation to the brain, I also have no final answers, but for many years now, I have been giving considerable thought to these topics. Unlike other tissues, the cells of the brain cannot replace themselves. They have lost the ability to reproduce. All Mr. Brohamer's neurons that were still functioning had been doing so for virtually all his seventy-seven years or more. And most would continue in that fashion. But like all of us, John Brohamer had been losing brain cells since he had reached age twenty or so. Not many—something like a few thousand a day. It's an element in the normal process of aging. Or is it really "normal?"

The death of neurons, which is part of everyday life, must be the result of one of two processes. The first possibility, which has been termed "programmed cell death," can be viewed as a flaw of cellular design. In specializing to do what they do so uniquely well, the neurons of the brain may have been designed to carry out those functions for only a finite length of time. If this is the case, then such cells are not built to last forever, and they gradually disappear as the years go by. Some last longer than do others, but the failure of these cells to survive is inherent in the cells themselves. Similarly, if this scenario is true, then senescence, that period of time during which functions are lost as the result of the passage of time, is inevitable whenever the life span has exceeded the projected life of the average individual cell. If this is the case, the answer to Mr. Brohamer's question depends upon learning whether those neurons that live to age seventy or eighty are any different biologically from those that die at age twenty. If they are, preventing senescence would depend on correcting the differences in those cells that are destined to die too soon, a task that may turn out to be the province of genetic engineers.

The second possibility conceives that neurons are designed to live forever. Each cell should then be capable of functioning for an infinite life span, but often our brains cells don't last that long. Why not? Perhaps ours don't live forever because of constant exposure to some sort of toxic factor that builds up slowly over the years, finally reaching levels that kill cells. Aging of the brain, then, is not really aging. It is merely the passage of time. The toxins begin to build up the day we are born. They reach "toxic" levels and begin to kill neurons at about age twenty. The year from seventy to seventy-one is no different from the year from twenty to twenty-one. Each is accomplished over 365 days. But what happens to the brain may well be different, since seventy years of continued exposure have preceded the former and only twenty the latter. In this scenario, prolonging the lives of the individual cells depends upon identifying and eliminating the toxins or finding some sort of antidote to prevent them from doing any further harm.

I took as careful a history from Mr. Brohamer as I could. I tried to determine whether he had ever suffered from any possible neurologic problem. Lead can cause degeneration of the peripheral nerves. Manganese can cause a state that is somewhat like parkinsonism. Toluene can cause cerebellar disease leading to ataxia. The list of possible toxins is long. The best way to start is to find the symptoms and then explore possible exposures to those toxins that can cause them.

He had no symptoms.

I started from the other direction. Did he have any known toxic exposure? At work? At home? In the garden? Pesticides are by design toxic. So are herbicides. In any other hobby?

Once again, I came up empty-handed.

But John Brohamer had not come to me concerned about symptoms. Rather, he wanted me to tell him how to avoid all the possible toxins of this world. What he wanted, in effect, was a universal antidote, which medical science has for years referred to as a mithridate. Physicians of the ancient world spent a great deal of time and energy attempting to design such concoctions. Centuries later, alchemists continued the same search—the endless quest for a "mithridate"—named after the first man who successfully designed and used one such formulation.

The Mithridates who invented the universal antidote was not an alchemist, but the king of the petty kingdom of Pontus in Asia Minor. He was the sixth and last king of his name to reign in Pontus [120–63 B.C.] and during his lifetime fought three protracted wars with Rome. Mithridates VI's fame rests not only on his ability to wage war relatively successfully against the Romans, but is a reflection of his interest in poisons and antidotes. His fascination with this subject began early in his life. While his mother was regent, he realized that she enjoyed power and would not easily relinquish it when he reached his majority. This story is reported by the Byzantine historian Justin, who wrote that Mithridates's guardians "tried to cut him off by poison. He, however, being on his guard against treachery, frequently took antidotes, and so fortified himself by exquisite preventives against their malice." Young Mithridates, it appears, noticed something was amiss; perhaps there was a queer taste to his food. In his circumstances, such a death was not an unlikely possibility. At the Pontic court, it seems, murder by slow poison had become such a matter of routine that it always followed the same course: One particular poison was employed in small cumulative doses, which were guaranteed to bring death with all the symptoms of natural disease. Some doctors, however, believed they had discovered an antidote to this poison, which the young prince took in a regular daily dose. In fact, he continued this regime until the day of his death some fifty years later. Each day after swallowing his mithridate, he would take a small dose of poison, to make sure that the antidote had been properly compounded. Once this routine was established, he found that he could eat without any ill effects the most elaborate recipes of the palace cooks.

Mithridates continued his study of poisons after he assumed the throne. He knew that more than one poison existed and that to be safe, he would need more than just one antidote. Of the ancient medical authors, Galen had the greatest interest in pharmacology and in mithridates. In the opening part of his *De Antidotis,* Galen stated that Mithridates was zealous to have empirical or experimental knowledge of almost all the simple drugs that could be used to combat poisons. To obtain this information, Mithridates tested them on condemned criminals. Through such experimentation, he found some drugs that were effective against the poison of spiders, some against scorpions, and others against vipers. Other agents appeared to counteract lethal poisons, from aconite and sea slugs. By mixing all these agents together, Mithridates created a single medication that he hoped would offer protection against all poisons. Subsequently, Andromachus, by adding several ingredients and removing others, prepared the antidote called theriac, which included a considerable amount of the flesh of vipers, a component absent from the original mithridate. Without any experimental data but only this theoretical basis, Galen believed that theriac was better for viper bites than was the mithridate. Later, he presented actual recipes for making the mithridate and another antidote known as a panacea.

How successful was the original mithridate? Perhaps the story of the death of Mithridates himself, as relayed to us by Plutarch, is the best evidence of the efficacy of his regimen. When his army was finally defeated by the Roman legions under Pompey the Great, Mithridates decided to kill himself with Pontic poison, which he had hidden in the pommel of his sword. First, he gave small doses to his two daughters, who begged to die with him. The drug took effect upon them at once, and they perished quickly and painlessly. They had never needed to take the antidote during their highly sheltered lives. The old king swallowed what was left in his sword-hilt and walked rapidly about the room, to encourage the poison to flow through his veins. But more than fifty years of the daily antidote had immunized his body, and the drug failed to affect him. At last he understood he could not die by poison. There was still among his following a nobleman named Bituitus, a chieftain of Galatia who had stood by his lord to the last. Mithridates turned to him, reminding him that for many years he had relied on his sharp sword and strong right arm: "But although I have been on my guard against all the poisons that a man may take with his food, I have neglected to provide against that most deadly, to be found in every royal palace: the treason of soldiers, of sons, and of friends." All other alternatives having failed, Mithridates ordered Bituitus to kill him. Obeying his liege to the last, Bituitus cut him down.

And Mr. Brohamer thought his request was a simple one. He had no signs or symptoms of excessive toxic exposure. That meant that there was no poison concentrated to an abnormal degree in his body that could be removed or counteracted to return him to normal health.

I told him that.

He did not take this information with any degree of equanimity. He told me that he already knew that, and besides, that had not been what he had wanted to learn when he decided to pay me a visit.

"What can you do about the normal toxins?" he asked.

Ten or fifteen years ago, I would have disregarded his question as meaningless. Today, things are different. We do not have any definite answers but, like Mr. Brohamer, we are at least beginning to ask the question. *Do* nerve cells actually die from toxic exposure?

Cells are constantly in need of repair, for life is a series of minor insults. In response to the nicks and scratches of day-to-day existence, our skin repairs itself, and each cell repairs itself, its membranes, its organelles, its mitochondria, its RNA, its proteins and enzymes, and its DNA, which controls the RNA. But DNA repair can fail, and if it does, the cell will die from the normal wear and tear that it can no longer correct.

What causes such wear and tear? Poisons. Toxins. Man-made chemicals, the plague of our atmosphere—of course.

But they cannot be the major culprits, and in fact, they may not even be a factor. In our highly polluted age, more people, and thereby more nerve cells, are living longer then ever. But there are also naturally occurring toxins. Most plants produce such chemicals, which repel insects and microbes. Most antibiotics, which kill off bacteria so successfully, are derived from other living cells. There is an untold number of such substances in the world, and they have been here forever. After all, aging and death are not new problems. Isn't it possible that these substances can slowly collect in the brain and even more slowly injure and then kill its neurons?

But how would they do so?

By oxidation. Some of the toxins act as unstable, chemically active molecules called free radicals. These free radicals attach themselves to the normal working parts of the cell; the RNA, the DNA, and the cell membranes, then oxidize these components, rendering them useless. As a result of this process, the membranes become leaky. The RNA, in turn, can no longer make membrane proteins or enzymes. The membranes become progressively weaker. The cell's metabolism slows down. The DNA can no longer direct the RNA or repair itself. Finally, the cell slows down and dies. The one-horse shay can no longer roll along the roadway, or even be dragged out of the stable. It has been oxidized. It has become so rusty that it is frozen in place.

How can we prevent such rusting? There is no simple answer. There are molecules that act an antioxidants. These scavengers could enter the brain, search out the free radicals, and inactivate them, thereby saving the cell from destruction and death. Such a molecule would be a drug manufacturer's dream come true, for every person in the world would take it every day, forever. Designing such a drug could cost billions, and it could take years. And it undoubtedly did. Such molecules, in fact, already exist and have been with us forever. The best studied one is Vitamin E.

When I was in medical school, vitamin E was barely mentioned. It was not even dignified by being accepted as a true vitamin. It was the only vitamin whose deficiency did not cause a disease. B-12 deficiency causes pernicious anemia; niacin deficiency, pellagra; vitamin C, scurvy; and so forth, until you got to so-called vitamin E. No deficiency state. No disease at all. How could it be a real vitamin? It couldn't. It wasn't.

That may no longer be the case.

Does vitamin E help preserve neurons? Does it keep any brain cells from dying? As of yet, we don't know for certain, but research is being conducted in this area. Our model is Parkinson's disease. Why Parkinson's disease? Because that disorder is caused by the selective death of cells of the substantia nigra, a collection of cells in the base of the brain that contain melanin. Melanin attracts free radicals, which, as they build up in the nerve cells of the substantia nigra, might well play a role in injuring and finally killing it. *If* this is true and *if* vitamin E could slow down this process, then vitamin E might slow down the rate at which the cells die, which is the rate at which Parkinson's disease progesses from a mild discomfort to a severely disabling disorder. (And vitamin E would finally have its own disease.)

A federally funded study is now being carried out in twenty centers across the country to investigate vitamin E, and ought to have results in three or four years.

Each day, my patients with Parkinson's disease ask me whether they should take vitamin E.

"It's like choosing whether to believe in God or not," I tell them. "If you choose not to believe in God and you find out after you die that there is a God and believing in him would have made a difference, it's too late to go back. If, four years from now, we find out it works, you can't go back."

"So I should take vitamin E?"

"That you have to decide for yourself."

"Would you, Doc?"

"Yes. But I believe in God."

Author's Note

The best summary of the life of Mithridates VI is in volume 9 of the Cambridge Ancient History, *The Roman Republic*, edited by J. B. Bury et al. (London: Cambridge University Press, 1971). Justin and Plutarch are quoted from here. The best ancient source is Appian, whose *History* is primarily a history of the wars of Rome, including the important Mithridatic Wars. Plutarch's lives of Sulla, Lucullus, and Pompeius all deal in part with Mithridates. Alfred Duggan's novel/biography *He Died Old, Mithridates Eupator, King of Pontus* (London: Peter Davies, 1958) is heartily recommended to anyone who can find a copy. Saul Jarcho has summarized much that is recorded by ancient historians and physicians about the pharmaceutical interests of Mithridates VI (*Bulletin of the New York Academy of Medicine* [1972]:48, 1059–63).

Since this chapter was completed, our entire perspective on the role of toxins in Parkinson's disease has undergone a revolution. It has now been shown that an enzyme inhibitor called deprenyl (Eldepryl or selerguline) can slow down the rate at which the disease progresses. This is the first time that that has been accomplished in the treatment of any "degenerative disease." Deprenyl does not improve anything. A patient who takes it feels no better. His tremor does not improve nor does his imbalance nor his slowness. Instead, the rate at which these symptoms would increase is retarded.

How does this happen? The exact answer is unknown. The theory is based upon the hypothesis that some unknown toxin plays a pivotal role in killing specific brain cells in Parkinson's disease and that in order to do its dirty work this poison must first be activated by the particular enzyme that deprenyl blocks. The report of the nationwide, multicenter study that demonstrated this was just completed and published. (Parkinson Study Group, "Effect of Deprenyl on the Progression of Disability in Early Parkinson's Disease," *New England Journal of Medicine* 321 [1989]: 1364–71). The role of vitamin E is still being studied.

14

Joshua's Curse

It isn't often that a biblical story helps a physician make a correct diagnosis of a patient, especially a patient he has never examined. It happened to me only once, and I doubt if it will ever happen again. And it wasn't even a neurologic disease, but an illness caused by a small parasite. It was the story of Joshua and the walls of Jericho that came tumbling down that allowed me to make the diagnosis in a patient whom I never met, and about whom all I knew was a few symptoms and the fact that she had traveled to Jericho.

One of the biggest problems with having a reputation as a diagnostician is that many people expect you to be able to make the correct diagnosis on a patient without ever seeing him or her. The process is not that easy. You need to get the history from the patient—the symptoms—and their progression. You must then examine the patient, after which you can build up a list of possible diagnoses, the differential diagnosis. But I am often called and told about a friend or a relative who is hundreds or thousands of miles away, then given a list of scattered facts, a symptom or two, and asked to decide what's wrong. I listen politely and refer them to a neurologist who is nearer and might actually get to examine the patient. But when it is the rabbi who calls, and it's his favorite niece, politeness is not sufficient.

It was early on a Thursday afternoon in September. I was in my office reviewing a questionnaire that one of my colleagues, Dr. Caroline M. Tanner, was designing to determine whether exposure to well water is one of the factors that contributed to Parkinson's disease. Well water as a risk factor for Parkinson's disease—And here I thought that well water was clean, was good for you.

What did I know? I'm just a city boy. But well water is standing water. Chemicals in the soil are leeched into it, and stay there—pesticides, herbicides, insecticides, what have you.

So I was already thinking about wells before I got the call from my rabbi, and he started to tell me about his niece.

He knew most of the basics. Not enough to make a formal presentation, but enough to get started.

She was twenty-one and had never been sick before. It had begun a month ago.

"What?" I asked, feeling I had to say something.

Diarrhea, weight loss, being tired all the time, pain in her abdomen, blood in her urine.

These were not neurologic problems, I told him.

He knew that. He was getting to her neurologic problem: Shooting pains. Where?

Starting in her back and radiating around her flank into her stomach.

That indeed was neurologic. We call it radicular pain, or root pain, and it is characterized by electric, shooting pains from irritation of a nerve root as it leaves the spinal cord to travel to that part of the skin it carries messages to and from. Any process that compresses or irritates a root causes such pain—literally anything. The list of potential sources is all but endless.

Any differential diagnosis I could make would be too long and contain too many possibilities. Without talking to her and examining her, it would be speculation, not diagnosis.

It could be anything, I told him.

Such as?

A tumor, a ruptured disc, an infection . . . I stopped myself. How old was she?

Twenty-one.

Did she go to college?

Yes. BU.

What?

Boston University, he explained to this uninitiated Midwesterner.

Where had she spent her junior year?

Israel.

Where in Israel?

Hebrew University. In Jerusalem.

Anywhere else?

She went all over Israel. It's a small country, as I well knew.

Had she been to Jericho?

Did it matter?

Yes.

He'd find out, he said, and hung up.

Jericho.

The well.

I hadn't thought about it in years—Jericho and its well and Joshua's curse on them both. So instead of pondering Dr. Tanner's wells, I turned my attention to Jericho's, better known as the Well of the Prophet Elisha. I have been to Jericho several times, each time starting my trip from Jerusalem.

The road from Jerusalem to Jericho begins just outside the walls of the Old City. It passes through the Kidron Valley, on the eastern edge of Jerusalem, below the Garden of Gethsemane whose olive trees were already too ancient in the seventh century for the Muslims to put a tax on them. The road winds through the valley to reach Bethany, a village on the southeastern slope of the Mount of Olives. In Arabic, this village is called El Azarinzeh, "the place of Lazarus." It was here that Jesus went, accompanied by his Apostles, and raised Lazarus from the dead. Beyond Bethany, the road turns toward the Dead Sea. Soon it is below sea level, and then, off to the left, lies Jericho—or, more correctly, the Jerichos, for there has been more than one Jericho in the past nine thousand years. Villages and cities have come and gone. Some have been built on top of previous ones. Others have carved out new territory. There are at least four separate Jerichos: ancient and biblical Jericho, Jericho of Herod's (and Jesus's) time, Arab Jericho of the eighth century, and modern Jericho.

I have seen all these Jerichos. I have seen remnants of those walls that came tumbling down. I have even visited the famous Well of Jericho blessed by the Prophet Elisha. But I did not drink the water from this well. Had the rabbi's niece? If she were my patient, I'd ask her directly.

Jericho is 900 feet below sea level in the deep valley of the river Jordan. It is about five miles west of the river and the same distance north of the Dead Sea. It is an oasis town, and wells supply it with water. Jericho is one of the oldest cities in the world. It existed as a walled city during the Stone Age, about 4,000 years ago. In spite of its favorable location and abundant water supply, the site was actually left uninhabited for some six hundred years, from 1300 B.C. to 700 B.C., give or take a few decades.

Why was it deserted then?

The Bible gives us one explanation, medicine a second. And the second merely amplifies the first. The second is a matter of science, the first, of faith.

The rabbi called back. His niece had been to Jericho. She had stayed there for several weeks in July, after her school year was over.

Doing what?

Digging at one of the archaeological sites.

Had she drunk from the well? I asked. I did not have to explain which well.

"Elisha's Well?" he asked.

"Of course."

He had no idea, but he'd find out.

I tried to go back to the protocol, but my mind remained riveted on Jericho and its well water. Jericho and the entry to the Promised Land. I opened my Bible, and glanced through the story, in the Book of Joshua.

After forty years of wandering in the desert, Joshua led the Israelites across the River Jordan and toward the fertile highlands of Judea. Jericho, strategically positioned along this route, was the first walled city that had to be conquered. As a preliminary step in this process, Joshua dispatched spies into the city, who were hidden by one of the natives of Jericho, a woman named Rahab. Although Rahab is often referred to euphemistically as an innkeeper, any accurate translation of the biblical Hebrew tells us that she was a prostitute. She eventually helped the spies to escape after extracting a promise of protection for herself and her family. The spies returned to Joshua confident that the city could be taken. After all, morale in Jericho was low, and the inhabitants expected to be conquered.

Joshua laid siege to Jericho and captured it. The biblical narrative tells how the walls of Jericho crumbled to give the Israelite army easy access to the city. Once Jericho fell, Joshua ordered all the inhabitants to be killed: men, women, children, and domestic animals. Only Rahab and her family were spared. Joshua then laid down a curse:

"Cursed before the Lord be the man that rises up and rebuilds this city, Jericho. At the cost of his first-born shall he lay its foundation, and at the cost of his youngest son shall he set up its gates."

The Bible says nothing more about Jericho for several hundred years. The next mention is in Kings, so I flipped the pages forward. During the reign of Ahab, Hiel of Bethel attempted to rebuild Jericho, but "he laid its foundation at the cost of Abiram his first-born, and set up its gates at the cost of his youngest son Segub, according to the word of the Lord which he spoke by Joshua the son of Nun."

Obviously Joshua's curse was working.

Finally, centuries later, in Second Kings, the Prophet Elisha was asked to cleanse the well of Jericho by men who wanted to settle there. "Behold the situation of this city is pleasant, as my Lord sees; but the water is bad, and the land unfruitful." In other English translations of the Bible, the Hebrew word for "unfruitful" is translated as "barren" or "childless," and the New English Bible uses an entirely different phrase: "The country was troubled with miscarriages."

Elisha did what they asked. By throwing some salt into the well, he cleansed it. So even today, the well in Jericho is known as Elisha's Well.

That's the entire biblical account, which raises more questions than it answers.

Why did the inhabitants of Jericho expect to be beaten by Joshua? Why did the walls of the city crumble so easily? Why did Joshua take the extraordinary step of annihilating the citizenry and their domesticated animals? Why did Jericho then remain deserted for centuries? And how did the infertility of the land and the people somehow tie up with the well—Elisha's Well?

And had the rabbi's niece drunk from that well?

Archaeological evidence helped to answer all but the last of these questions. The rabbi's niece herself could answer the final one.

Archaeology confirmed the biblical story: Jericho was actually deserted for several hundred years. And its walls, which crumbled so easily, were in fact made of mud bricks. The water for those bricks came out of Elisha's Well, and the bricks contain shells of a small snail known as *bulinus truncatus*.

And therein is the explanation for the entire story—and the reason why the rabbi's niece should have avoided Elisha's Well.

The phone rang again. It was the rabbi. He'd talked to his niece again. She had drunk water from the well.

"Schistosomiasis," I said.

"What?" he replied.

"Bulinus truncatus," I explained.

He was not impressed by my explanation.

Bulinus truncatus is a snail, I told him, that carries a disease known as schistosomiasis. Schistosomes are small parasites, whose life story is complicated. The parasites leave the water snail *bulinus truncatus* as free-swimming forms. They enter the human body by penetrating the skin and then pass into the circulation. After they have matured and mated in the veins of the liver, the female lays her eggs around the bladder. These eggs work their way through the bladder wall and are passed in the urine. If they then enter fresh water, each egg ruptures, releasing a microscopic parasite that enters *bulinus truncatus* and completes the life cycle by developing into a more mature form that can then infect the next human who drinks the water.

"My niece?"

"Yes. The blood in her urine."

"That was several weeks ago."

"That was the eggs going through the wall of her bladder and . . ."

"I understand," he protested. He didn't need all the gruesome details. "Are you sure she has schistosome-whatsis?"

Of course I wasn't.

"She looks healthy."

"Most people do," I replied.

Patients with mild infections usually have few signs and symptoms, but repeated contact with infected water increases the number of parasites in the body and leads to severe infections. When this happens, other organs become involved, and patients suffer complications like urinary obstruction; anemia; weight loss; wasting; and, more important, impotence in men and sterility in women.

"My niece?" he interrupted.

"Rahab," I countered.

"Barrenness," he recalled. "Does it do that?"

"And impotence," I reminded him.

"And who," the rabbi countered, "could have been in a better position than Rahab the prostitute to evaluate whether schistosomiasis had spread among the men of Jericho and caused an epidemic of impotence?"

I resisted the temptation to credit her with first-hand evidence.

"It explains the entire story of Jericho," I continued. The walls of Jericho, I reminded him, were made of mud bricks. Such walls are in need of constant repair. If schistosomiasis were epidemic in Jericho, it might explain why the walls tumbled down so easily. Listlessness and apathy are common in patients with schistosomiasis. That could have made them careless, so that they may have failed to repair the city walls. The Israelites had no such illness, and thus were more than a match for the debilitated inhabitants of Jericho. Serious, chronic ill health in a community might certainly lower morale and explain the defeatist attitude of its inhabitants.

How about Elisha and the cleansing of the well?

The best way to prevent schistosomiasis is to destroy the intermediate host, the snail in which it completes its life cycle. *Bulinus truncatus* lives only in fresh water. A change in climate, such as a prolonged drought, could easily result in the disappearance of the snail. And there are many biblical references to drought during the time when Jericho was abandoned. *Bulinus truncatus* cannot completely seal its shell. This makes it particularly sensitive to periods of excessive dryness. Hence, the well at Jericho could have been cleared of *bulinus truncatus* by a period of drought.

So perhaps Elisha did not cleanse the well after all.

The handful of salt that Elisha cast into the water when requested to cleanse the well would not kill off the snails. Presumably, *bulinus truncatus* was no longer present, and Elisha was merely carrying out a ritual purification to reassure the populace.

"Elijah," the rabbi said.

"What?"

"Elijah. He was Elisha's predecessor and prophet in residence, and during Elijah's life, there was a severe drought that lasted three years."

"I forgot that," I said, assuming that I had once known it.

He hung up.

There were, as far as I knew, no further biblical complaints about the conditions at Jericho, and presumably the district prospered. When Cleopatra wanted Judea as part of her domain, her consort, Mark Anthony, tried to protect the throne of his friend Herod the Great by giving Cleopatra the revenues of some of the richest areas in the region, among which was Jericho. Jericho is mentioned a number of times in the Gospels and, according to contemporary records, flourished in the Byzantine and early Muslim eras.

The rabbi called again. "Her pain?" he asked. "What's causing that?"

"Schistosomiasis," I replied.

"How?"

"The eggs are causing irritation of the nerve roots as they travel through the body."

"Ah," he said.

Two days later, the rabbi called me. His niece's doctor, in Portland, had made the diagnosis. And as far as the rabbi knew, that doctor had never even been to Jericho. He was an internist who specialized in infectious diseases and was a good physician.

I didn't ask if her doctor had ever heard of Joshua's curse.

"What should we do?" he asked.

"About your niece? Nothing. She's in good hands."

"No, she's fine. But what should we do about the well?"

"Call Elisha. Or, better yet, you should go there and throw in some salt and repeat the same prayers that Elisha said."

The rabbi thought it would be more effective if he called a friend of his who had a nephew who worked in Israel's Ministry of Health. The rabbi has always been a practical man.

Author's Note

Although the theory that schistosomiasis is the medical basis for Joshua's curse and the subsequent abandonment of Jericho goes back to H. E. Biggs's "Mollusca from Prehistoric Jericho" (*Journal of Conchology* [1970]:24,379). it has been most fully documented and explained by E. V. Hulse (*Medical History* [1978]:23,14–26). Fortunately, I had read this before the rabbi called me about his niece. Much of the argument used here was first presented by Hulse.

=15=

The Subject at Risk

What inspiration I have goes into getting it not quite right in the first place.
—Simon Gray, An Unnatural Pursuit

The question that she asked was one that I had been asked before, more than once. I had not known how to answer it the other times, and I still didn't know when Harriet Steinfeldt posed it to me. She worded it much more articulately than any of the other patients had, using much more precise and scientifically accurate terms. Her succinct way of phrasing it, however, did not increase my ability to supply her with a reasonable answer.

Ms. Steinfeldt was the eldest daughter of a patient of mine. She was one of six children who ranged in age from twelve to twenty-three. Her father, Harvey, had been my patient since I had been a second-year neurology resident—a period of only three years. Harvey Steinfeldt had Huntington's chorea, a hereditary disease of the brain causing abnormal movements (chorea), personality changes, and dementia. He had inherited the gene that carries that disease from his mother. She, in turn, had received it from her mother, who had also inherited it from someone. Whom, I either never knew or no longer recall. I didn't bother to record it in Harry's chart; I'm not a genealogist, and going back more than two generations makes no difference to me as a treating physician.

Huntington's chorea is always hereditary and it's always inherited as an autosomal dominant trait. That means that each child of a parent with the disease has a fifty-fifty chance of inheriting the gene and the disease that comes with the gene. There are no "carriers." Every person who has the gene—and, therefore, has the capability of passing that gene on to members of the next generation—sooner or later develops the disorder. As physician/scientists, we call each offspring of a patient with Huntington's chorea a "subject at risk" for the disease. Harriet was, unquestionably, a "subject at risk."

The symptoms of Huntington's chorea almost always begin after age thirty, sometimes as late as fifty or fifty-five, and occasionally even later. Because of this delayed onset, subjects at risk of Huntington's chorea are still free of any hint of disease during that time of life when most of their offspring are conceived and born. This had been true of Harriet's father. His symptoms had first appeared when he was thirty-eight. Harriet had been conceived when he was twenty. When Harriet's youngest brother was born, their father was only thirty-two and was robust, healthy, and without a care in the world, other than supporting his wife and family, which he did quite well. Here lies the dilemma: Those who are destined to develop Huntington's chorea—and who are thereby capable of passing the gene and the disease on to the next generation—cannot be told apart from their siblings who are normal and will never develop the disease and therefore cannot and will not transmit it to their offspring. Because of this, there is no way to offer reasonable genetic counseling to those who are at risk for Huntington's chorea.

That was Harriet's question. She asked it right out. "I'm a subject at risk for Huntington's chorea," she said. "I want to know what my children's chances would be of getting the disease."

She already knew her chances. Hers were 50:50: 1 out of 2. Statistically, her children's chances were half that: 25:75, 1 out of 4, 25 percent. But that figure is a lie, a statistical lie. It's true that 25 percent of all the children conceived and born in that situation would develop Huntington's chorea. But not one of those children really has a 25 percent chance. Each has either a 50 percent chance—if the parent at risk had the abnormal gene—or a 0 percent chance—if the parent at risk did not possess the gene.

That much she already knew. What she came to ask me was whether I could tell her to which group she belonged. Not for her sake—she had already resigned herself to the fact that she might develop the disease, and knew that die had been cast long ago—but for the sake of her yet-unconceived children and grandchildren.

I had no way to answer her question, and I told her as much. She, in turn, asked me to keep her in mind and to call her if we ever did have an answer. I told her that I would, but, I doubted that I'd ever make that call or that I would ever give this conversation another thought. Science moves much more slowly than those who are not involved in it realize.

That afternoon, I tried to answer another, far different question. There was some travel money left over in one of my research grants. If I could locate a worthwhile scientific meeting in a reasonable place at the right time of the year, I could spend these funds and have an enjoyable vacation at the same time. I wanted to go to Europe, and the only free time I had would be in August. The only conference that looked all that interesting was a meeting of the World Federation of Neurology Research Group on Huntington's chorea. The organization was headed by André Barbeau, a neurologist from Montreal whom I had met several times. He was one of the few international figures in the field of Parkinson's disease who went out of his way to befriend and assist younger investigators. Most of the others seemed to view their junior colleagues as potential threats. Since I was in that category then, I very much appreciated André's support.

So I called André and asked him about the conference, expressing my interest in being invited to participate.

He told me that it was a small meeting of investigators who had a dedicated interest in Huntington's chorea. I was welcome to attend if I considered myself to fall in that category.

"Would I ask to be invited if I didn't?" I asked, with the brashness of youth. Not exactly a lie, but pretty close. I was interested in Huntington's chorea. It was not just a passive interest, but, then again, I had done no actual research.

It was good enough for André, trusting soul that he was, and invited me to attend.

That night, what I had done hit me.

"Dedicated to the study of Huntington's chorea." I figured that I'd better get started working on some aspect of the disease, but which one? That was obvious. There was only one area that I wanted to investigate.

Harriet's question.

"I'm a subject at risk for Huntington's chorea," she had said. "I want to know what my children's chances would be of getting the disease."

Where to start?

That much I already knew. I had not totally lied to André. I cared about Huntington's chorea, both about the patients and their problems and about the disease itself. The subject had fascinated me since I'd been a medical student. I'd read much of the medical literature; it was time to reread it.

I began by asking myself a simple question, What causes chorea? Not the disease, Huntington's chorea, but the abnormal movements that are called chorea. The word *chorea* is derived from the Greek word for dance and was originally applied to describe the dancelike gait and continual limb movements seen in the dancing mania—a hysterical disease of the fifteenth century. The term *chorea* is now applied to describe a class of abnormal spontaneous movements, each of which is a single, isolated muscle action—a short, rapid, uncoordinated jerk. These jerks can be located in any muscle, causing that part of the body to move in an unpredictable way. The successive occurrence of two or more such isolated jerks can result in more complicated movements, while the superimposition of normal movements on top of these abnormal ones can cause complex movement patterns, such as the classic dancelike gait.

These abnormal movements are the most characteristic manifestation of Huntington's chorea. They occur in almost all patients and are frequently the first complaint. Harry Steinfeldt had had such abnormal movements, and so had his mother. It was the movements that had made him come to see me for a diagnosis. Harriet had not experienced this symptom—at least not yet.

Why do patients with Huntington's chorea get chorea? What brain mechanism underlies the chorea, causing the abnormal movement to take place?

I read everything I could find on the subject. As far as I could tell, the exact mechanism that initiates the abnormal movements in Huntington's chorea was not clear to anyone. Several authorities attributed the movements to the absence of the normal filter mechanism of the diseased striatum, the area of the brain most affected by the process of Huntington's chorea. These theories were difficult, if not impossible, to interpret in terms of biochemistry or cellular physiology.

It was this interface of chemistry and physiology that intrigued me. If there is a chemical change in the brain, how does it produce chorea? The discovery of decreased levels of dopamine in patients who died of parkinsonism and the subsequent successful use of L-dopa in the treatment of that disease had revolutionized our understanding of Parkinson's disease in only a few years. Perhaps the same could be done for Huntington's chorea.

Like everyone else, I, too, believed that the abnormal movements in Huntington's chorea were related to the pathologic changes in the striatum. Whatever the gene does in Huntington's chorea, it does to the cells of this part of the brain: The neurons that make up the striatum progressively die off as a result of the genetic defect. Then-current theory held that the loss of these calls led to chorea. But there was another possibility: Chorea might be related to the abnormal function of diseased, but, still living, neurons. This is more than a subtle difference. It might prove far easier to treat symptoms due to the abnormal behavior of living cells than any due to a loss of function caused by cell death. Chorea could be caused by some neurochemical such as dopamine acting on the diseased striatal neurons. What made this hypothesis particularly attractive to me was the distinct possibility that this approach might help answer Harriet's question.

All I needed was a little bit of luck.

Why had I picked on dopamine? Dopamine is not the only neurotransmitter that acts upon the striatum—there are several others. Also, it was not just because I knew a lot about dopamine. It was because what I knew about it made it the best candidate. There was already plenty of evidence that dopamine was related to the production of chorea. I did not discover this information. Neurologists knew how to treat patients with Huntington's and to control the chorea. It was my belief that if I knew how to control a function of the brain [chorea] with a drug and I knew how that drug worked, then, of necessity, I knew something about the mechanism behind that behavior. Agents such as chlorpromazine (Thorazine) and haloperidol (Haldol), which had originally been introduced and are still widely used to treat schizophrenia, also ameliorate chorea. These drugs work by blocking the dopamine receptors (the parts of the nerve call that respond to dopamine) on the striatal neurons. Other drugs like reserpine, which decrease the level of dopamine in the striatum, had also been shown to improve chorea.

If drugs that block or decrease the activity of dopamine in the striatum decrease the severity of chorea, then it would seem reasonable that in some way, dopamine caused chorea. How could that come to pass? The first possibility was that the amount of dopamine in the brain could be increased in Huntington's chorea. The evidence in the medical literature suggested that this was not the case. The same investigators who showed that dopamine was decreased in Parkinson's disease studied dopamine in Huntington's chorea and found that the concentration of dopamine in the striatum was normal.

If dopamine levels are normal, how, then, could dopamine have any relation to something as obviously abnormal as chorea?

There was one possible answer. Since the concentration of dopamine is normal in patients with Huntington's chorea, the response of the nerve cells to this normal amount of dopamine itself would have to be abnormal. Why? Huntington's leaves the cells that contain the dopamine receptors diseased and dying. Thus, it seemed reasonable to hypothesize that diseased cells have abnormal receptors and that a hypersensitive or increased response of these dopamine receptors of the striatum to the normal amounts of dopamine is responsible for the appearance of abnormal movements in this disease.

This was a completely different way of looking at chorea itself: Chorea was not due to the loss of function of dead striatal neurons, but to the abnormal function of diseased neurons. It was a new theory, but would it help Harriet Steinfeldt?

It just might. If altered responsiveness to normal amounts of dopamine proved to be the cause of chorea, it might be possible to bring out the chorea in subjects at risk while they were still at that stage by increasing the amount of dopamine in their brains.

My logic went something like this. When he reached age thirty-seven or so, normal levels of dopamine acting deep inside Harvey Steinfeldt's brain began to cause chorea because his brain, or more specifically, the dopamine receptors of his brain, responded in an abnormal way. The genetic defect that caused that abnormal response had been part of his makeup since inception. Yet the movements started only at age thirty-seven.

It was unlikely that suddenly, as if by magic, the receptors went from completely normal to distinctly abnormal, I thought. The symptoms certainly don't. The first symptoms of Huntington's chorea are often extremely subtle and may consist of just slight clumsiness or restlessness, associated later with overt twitching of the fingers and grimacing of the face. Early in the course of the disease, the abnormal movements may be seen only during attempts to maintain a limb in a sustained posture. As the disease progresses, however, the chorea becomes more and more striking and, eventually, all the patient's musculature is involved. The full-blown clinical picture includes not only facial grimacing (involving the lips, tongue, and cheeks) but jerks of the head, weaving movements of the arms and shoulders, and twists and jerks of the body—as well as superimposed voluntary movements carried out by the patient to hide the otherwise obvious involuntary movements. An upward jerk of an arm may be fused into a voluntary scratching of the head. The patient is virtually a stage on which numerous uncoordinated muscle movements take place. The patient's gait is often markedly involved. It is made up of jerky, lurching steps that are the result of a combination of voluntary and involuntary movements.

I had seen this sort of progression time and time again. I had observed it in Harvey Steinfeldt, and so had his family. To me, it seemed logical to assume that the receptor-site abnormality, like the chorea it caused, was not a yes/no, present/absent dichotomy, but a slow continuum. That meant that it was possible that slight degrees of abnormality were present long before any chorea occurred—perhaps years before. During those years, Harvey Steinfeldt had seemed normal. His behavior had been unexceptional, but his brain had begun its slow descent into disease. It seemed possible to me that the "abnormality" Huntington's caused could be uncovered by increasing the activity of dopamine within the brain of subjects at risk. If normal amounts of dopamine acting at very abnormal receptors caused chorea, then increased amounts acting on partially abnormal receptors might also cause chorea. All you had to do to see if this was true was to increase the level of dopamine in the brain of someone who had the gene but was still normal. And all you had to do to increase dopamine activity in the brain was to give L-dopa. The ability of L-dopa to enter the brain and be converted into dopamine is the basis of its value in treating Parkinson's disease.

This approach might someday give an answer to Harriet's question. The hypothesis assumed that L-dopa would not elicit chorea in normal persons and that, in asymptomatic subjects at risk, two populations could be identified: those in whom L-dopa produces chorea, and those in whom it does not. It would be supposed that the former would be presymptomatic patients, whereas the latter would be either normal siblings or patients with potential abnormal striatal cells that were not altered sufficiently to respond abnormally to L-dopa at the time of administration.

My logic could be diagrammed this way:

	DOPAMINE ACTIVITY	DOPAMINE RECEPTORS	CHOREA
Normal Subject	Normal	Normal	None
Subject at Risk Who Is Destined to Get Huntington's Chorea			
1. Normal conditions	Normal	Partially abnormal	None
2. L-dopa load	Increased	Partially abnormal	Chorea (if the receptors are abnormal enough)
Subject at Risk Who Is Not Destined to Get Huntington's Chorea			
1. Normal conditions	Normal	Normal	None
2. L-dopa load	Increased	Normal	None

I called Harriet Steinfeldt, who was now Harriet Evers. Her question had not been an idle one. I told her that I still did not have an answer, but at least I knew what question to ask, what study to carry out. I explained to her what I proposed to do. I wanted to give her L-dopa to see if she developed abnormal movements. I also wanted to give it to her husband to make sure that the assumption that normal people did not develop chorea from L-dopa was a correct one.

She wanted to know in practical terms precisely what she would learn from the study.

I had no idea.

Would it answer her question?

I could make no guarantees—none at all. I told her that I thought that we would learn something more about Huntington's chorea. We might discover if dopamine receptor-site abnormalities were present very early in the disease.

What about her question?

I hedged.

She still persisted.

If you get chorea, I told her, I think your chances are much more than 50:50.

"And if I don't?"

"Then they are probably less. How much less, I have no idea."

That was all I ever told her. I swear to that.

I gave her and her husband L-dopa.

They took the drug for two months. I saw them every week, and neither she nor he ever developed chorea.

She was one of thirty patients I, along with André Barbeau of the University of Montreal and George Paulson of Ohio State University studied in these tests.

Our results looked this way:

> Subjects at risk: 30
>> Chorea on L-dopa: 10 (33 percent)
>> No chorea on L-dopa: 20 (67 percent)
> Controls tested: 24
>> Chorea on L-dopa: 0
>> No chorea on L-dopa: 24

It is clear from these data that the use of L-dopa in subjects at risk for Huntington's chorea did define two separate populations. Abnormal movements (positive test) developed in the first group of ten subjects at risk, but not in the second (negative test). Two such groups did not exist in the control population: None of the twenty-four controls manifested chorea. This fact should not be interpreted to mean that L-dopa cannot ever produce chorea in a normal central nervous system, but it does suggest that, in the doses administered at these levels and given over a short time, L-dopa does not produce abnormal movements in normal subjects.

I and my associates were very cautious in our interpretation of the data from that study. A positive test did not necessarily prove that the patient had or would necessarily develop Huntington's chorea. What it did indicate was that the central nervous systems of the patients who tested positive differed from the brains of normal persons in their responses to a given dose of L-dopa. This finding might be highly suggestive that these subjects actually possessed the gene for Huntington's chorea. Only longitudinal studies would ever indicate the degree of accuracy of the prediction.

A negative test was less meaningful, since it was quite possible that at the time of the test, the subject's receptor sites were abnormal but not yet sufficiently abnormal to produce chorea. The patient may well have a negative test (falsely negative) at one point in time and a positive test at a second, later time when the necessary degree of alteration has occurred in the striatum.

These were the data on Huntington's chorea that I presented at the meeting of the World Federation of Neurology Research Group the following summer.

I didn't see Harriet again for eight years. I tracked her down to see what had happened to her as part of a follow-up study of all the patients from our original L-dopa experiment.

She was now thirty-one, and normal. She had no evidence of chorea, and she had three children. She was eternally grateful to me.

Why?

Because I had changed her life.

"How?" I asked.

"By telling me I would not get it. That way I could have children. You made it all possible. I was going to have my tubes tied."

"But I never told you that."

"Yes, you did," she insisted.

"No," I said. "I only said your chances were less than 50:50."

I had never said that she wouldn't get Huntington's. I'd merely said that her chances were probably less than 50 percent. I couldn't figure out how she could have possibly misunderstood me. Had I misled her? Had I not said what I meant to say. The test could still prove to be wrong. Those kids could themselves be subjects at risk. How could this have happened? All too easily, I'm afraid. The misinterpretation of what I had said to her was part of human nature. While I was interested in the theoretical basis of chorea, all she wanted to know was whether or not she was going to get the disease. When I didn't say that the test was positive; she knew it was negative and negative meant only one thing. She was safe. Her children would be safe. And so would their children be. Unto the seventh generation, if not more. I hope she was right.

The L-dopa provocative test for Huntington's chorea has come and gone. We never advocated its widespread use. We had no data on false positives and false negatives.

Our last follow-up was published in 1980. These were our results:

Subjects at risk: 30

Chorea on L-dopa: 10

Diagnosis of Huntington's chorea 8 years later: 5 (50 percent)

No chorea on L-dopa: 20

Diagnosis of Huntington's chorea 8 years later: 1 (5 percent)

So false negatives did occur. At least one subject at risk who failed to develop chorea when given L-dopa later went on to have Huntington's. Would Harriet be a second one?

Not yet: She is now thirty-seven.

Here's hoping.

Today we are well on the way to eliminating such guesswork, not by causing chorea in subjects at risk, but by studying the chromosomes of the families who carry Huntington's chorea. We now know that the gene for Huntington's chorea is on chromosome number four, and our ability to detect that gene is getting better every month. Eventually, a few simple blood samples studied by skilled geneticists will give a far more accurate answer.

That will not be the end of the problem. About two years after we published our first study about the preclinical detection of Huntington's, I was interviewed by a writer working for *The Smithsonian*. "I heard," she began, "that all the subjects with positive results committed suicide."

"That certainly will make long term follow-up difficult," I replied. By that time I was sick and tired of those rumors. No one had committed suicide. And, of course, that's the problem—telling a patient that he or she is definitely going to develop a progressive, debilitating, uniformly fatal neurological disease sometime in the next twenty years or so. Predicting who will get the disease may result in fewer patients in the next generation, but it does nothing for the present generation. To do something for them, identification of the gene must be followed by discovery of the defect caused by the gene and a way to reverse that defect. That will be the end. Hopefully, we are approaching the beginning of that end.

Author's Note

The two articles on L-dopa and the presymptomatic detection of Huntington's chorea are H. L. Klawans, G. W. Paulson, S. P. Ringel, and A. Barbeau, "Use of L-dopa in the Detection of Presymptomatic Huntington's Chorea," *New England Journal of Medicine*, 286 (1972):1332-34; and H. L. Klawans, C. G. Goetz, and S. Perlick, "Presymptomatic and Early Detection of Huntington's Disease," *Annals of Neurology*, 8 (1980): 343-47.

Gene detection in Huntington's chorea is one of the hottest fields of genetic research. The best recent summaries of our scientific knowledge of Huntington's chorea, including the exciting story of locating the gene, are J. B. Martin and J. F. Gusella, "Huntington's Disease," *New England Journal of Medicine* 315 (1986): 1267-75; and T. C. Gilliam, J. F. Gusella, and H. Lehrach, "Molecular Genetic Stratagies to Investigate Huntington's Disease," *Advances in Neurology* 48 (1987): 17-29.

=16=

She Could Have Danced All Night

In ballet a complicated story is impossible to tell . . . we can't dance synonyms.
—George Balanchine

Despite a wealth of detail and an overall complexity that may take years to master, the process of making a neurologic diagnosis is always the same. The patient comes to the neurologist with a problem. In medical parlance, this problem is referred to as the chief complaint (CC, in medical shorthand). The CC should trigger a list of possible causes, the differential diagnosis (DD). The rest of the patient's history, especially the history of the present illness (HPI), the neurologic exam (NE), and the entire workup should narrow the DD down to a single diagnosis (Dx).

It is only the details that differ from patient to patient, from CC to CC. If the CC is a seizure, the DD is extensive, and unless the HPI suggests a specific Dx, the workup may be both extensive and expensive, including such acronyms as EEG, CAT, and NMR, not to mention EMG (electromyogram), BAERs (brainstem auditory evoked responses), and even some tests for which there are no acronyms. If the CC is a tremor, the DD is far shorter, and the Dx will depend primarily on the HPI and NE. The front sheet prepared by my receptionist includes a place for the CC. When I first pick up the chart of a new patient, I read that CC and instantly formulate a potential DD.

That did not happen the first time I picked up Josette De Maestri's chart. I got no further than her name, and I knew the diagnosis. De Maestri is not a common name, at least not in Chicago. I had had three other patients by that name, two brothers and a sister. All three had had the same disease, Huntington's chorea. And one of them had had a daughter named Josette. She'd been about thirteen or fourteen then, but that was ten years earlier. So that Josette De Maestri had to be about twenty-three or twenty-four today. How many Josette De Maestris could there be?

This Josette De Maestri was twenty-four.

It had to be the same person, the daughter of my patient with Huntington's chorea. Huntington's is always hereditary. That meant that Josette had a 50:50 chance of developing the disease.

She had not come to see me because of a CC. She had a chief question, "Do I have Huntington's chorea?"

And my DD was not a list of alternative possibilities. It was an all-or-none alternative. Either yes or no.

I looked at her sitting in the reception room and saw the brief jerks of chorea dart across her body. First her right shoulder shook, then her lips, then her left leg. Her lips twitched again, but not the same exact movement.

I continued to watch her; she continued to twitch.

I knew.

The answer was yes. She had Huntington's chorea.

And I was certain she already knew, as did her mother, who was sitting next to her.

Josette told me that she had been becoming increasingly nervous and agitated for the past two years. She had always been "high strung," but her nervousness had been getting worse. But she thought she had discovered the source of her agitation: It was the neighbors; they were trying to poison her. Her paranoid belief had been developing over the previous six months, so that what began as a vague suspicion had become frank paranoia. And paranoid ideation is often one of the manifestations of Huntington's chorea.

Her mother had been aware of the abnormal movements for the past year or so.

I examined Josette, and the NE added very little. I told them the diagnosis, confirming what they both already suspected. Josette had Huntington's chorea. It was the Huntington's that had caused the change in her, the abnormal movements and now the paranoid ideas.

Her mother accepted my assessment, but Josette herself accepted only the first two notions. The neighbors *were* trying to kill her—with poison and rays.

It was her paranoia that was the problem, not the chorea itself. Josette called the police several times a day and complained about the neighbors.

She'd also phoned the FBI and the CIA— It was the Arabs who were behind it all.

She called the sheriff's office, and the Treasury Department, and even the postal inspectors—urging them to look for poisoned letters.

Something had to be done.

I put her on the antipsychotic agent Stelazine. Stelazine, a first cousin of Thorazine (chlorpromazine), the first successful antipsychotic drug, has been shown to be helpful in patients with Huntington's chorea. I started her on a small dose. In the next month, I had to increase the dosage twice, but then she began to improve. Her paranoia disappeared. The chorea, her various twitches and jerks, improved. She even became less agitated.

Her mother was pleased, and so was Josette. So were the neighbors—to say nothing of the police and the postal inspectors.

Then, three months later, her mother called me. Josette was worse. She didn't want to go to sleep at night. That had been one of her earlier symptoms: When she'd been sure the neighbors were trying to kill her, she'd refused to go to sleep for fear they would sneak up and pour poison in her car. And she'd insisted that the radio had to stay on, otherwise the neighbors would send rays through it.

Had she said anything about the neighbors this time?

No.

Any paranoid ideas?

No.

Anything about poisons?

No.

About the rays? Or the radio?

No.

Had she called the police?

No.

Just the agitation and a refusal to go to bed.

I increased the Stelazine.

The agitation got worse. She insisted that the radio had to stay on all night. She said nothing about poisons or rays, but had begun to pace about anxiously at night.

More Stelazine.

More pacing, and she played the radio even more loudly.

I switched her to a more powerful antipsychotic drug: Haldol.

The pacing continued.

More Haldol.

She played the radio even louder, and began to dance.

More Haldol.

She danced all night.

This time it was the neighbors who called the police. The noise of Josette's radio had kept them awake.

The police came to the De Maestri house, and at nine in the morning they deposited Josette in my office. I talked to her for the first time in a month; all my previous telephone conversations had been with her mother. Josette paced back and forth in the examining room and answered my questions without once breaking stride.

She was entirely rational.

She knew that no one wanted to poison her. No one could send rays through a radio, that was crazy.

Why was she pacing?

Because she had to move all the time.

Why had she danced all night?

It was more fun than pacing. With that she began to waltz.

It was not Huntington's chorea that had caused this crisis. She was not suffering from increasing paranoid psychosis from her disease. This problem I had caused. Josette had what we call akathisia, a need to move continually about. It's the twentieth-century version of the dancing mania, one of the two great plagues of the fifteenth and sixteenth centuries. The original dancing mania was a singular disorder that many contemporaries believed was caused by supernatural forces, although some maintained that it was caused by the bite of a tarantula. Josette's dancing mania was due neither to any supernatural forces nor a spider bite. It was caused by the medications I had given her. Akathisia is a side effect of antipsychotic drugs like Stelazine and Haldol. I had failed to make the correct Dx when her symptoms had recurred and begun a vicious cycle, increasing the dosage of her antipsychotic medication in an attempt to treat a psychosis that didn't exist. She still had Huntington's, but everything that happens to a patient with Huntington's does not have to be due to the Huntington's. That is a lesson I've never forgotten.

More medicine caused increased symptoms.

These symptoms were again misinterpreted, and led to my prescribing an even higher dosage, which caused a further increase in symptoms, until I finally saw the patient and recognized what had happened.

It is a trap that is all too easy to fall into, and I fell into it hook, line and sinker.

Akathisia.

The dancing mania.

They are probably not exactly the same.

———

From the twelfth to the fifteenth century, Europe was visited by a series of frightful plagues that scarcely gave its exhausted populace any time to recover. Smallpox ravaged the Continent, and measles was far more destructive than it is today. Leprosy abounded, and those afflicted with it were torn from their families and banished from society. Saint Anthony's fire, now all but forgotten, was the dread of town and country. This withering, deforming disease, which struck without warning, left behind it cruelly crippled bodies. Such tragic events were the accepted lot of life and were borne with remarkable resignation.

Then another scourge appeared, an illness far worse than any of the others: the bubonic plague, the infamous Black Death. It was an epidemic of unprecedented proportions that broke over Europe in a great wave. Entire villages were exterminated. Fields became neglected. Soon famine complicated the pestilence. And just as the plague receded and the population and economy began to recover, another wave struck.

From 1119 to 1340—a period of 221 years—the plague ravaged Italy, for example, sixteen times. No words can fully describe its horrors, but the people who witnessed them, who lived in those days so full of the uncertainty of life, of sorrow, and of anxiety, were driven to the point of hysteria.

It was at that point that the dancing mania began and spread like a contagion. Today, most historians view this phenomenon as a form of mass hysteria.

In 1374 a group of men and women who had come from Germany wandered into the streets of Aix-la-Chapelle. The members of the band formed a circle and then began to dance. They danced wildly, screaming with fury, foaming at the mouth, with all control over their senses lost. Finally, after many hours, they fell to the ground in exhaustion. In a short time, this disease spread to the spectators, who joined in the wild dances. It was soon carried to neighboring villages and from them outward in an ever-widening circle.

By 1418, this turmoil reached its highest point in the city of Strasbourg. Those afflicted could be seen dancing day and night, accompanied through the streets by musicians. By then, it was believed that music was a remedy, since the playing of music seemed, at times, to relieve the mass hysteria.

The other major epidemic of the same period was syphilis, and like syphilis, this was a new disease. In contrast to the base origin of syphilis, most contemporaries believed that the dancing mania had a superhuman origin and that the victims of this scourge could only be saved by the intervention of Saint Vitus, whose name became associated with the contagion. Patients often traveled to southern France, to the Tomb of Saint Vitus, to be cured. This pilgrimage was often made by groups of dancers, who spread their contagion as they traveled toward a possible cure. Paracelsus, the greatest physician of the period, became particularly interested in this phenomenon and he strenuously protested against this or any other disease being attributed to the devil or being named after a saint. Despite his usual rejection of ancient authorities, he accepted the rational reasoning of Hippocrates and insisted that all diseases could be ascribed to natural causes. He likewise rejected the notion that the intervention of Saint Vitus could cure this affliction. In place of invoking superhuman forces, Paracelsus devised his own harsh but effective treatment for the dancing mania. He subjected the victims of this apparent form of mass hysteria to such heroic measures as immersion in cold water, fasting, and solitary confinement. As his therapeutic approach gained acceptance, the hysterical outbreaks of the dancing mania began to subside. Whether the cure itself or the threat of it encouraged the cessation of these peculiar dances is a question that is still unanswered.

Traditional medical wisdom teaches us that the dancing mania was a form of mass hysteria. I once accepted that wisdom unquestioningly, but I am no longer as certain as I once was. My experience with patients like Josette De Maestri has made me newly skeptical.

Josette's dancing was not a form of hysteria and it was not related to any type of psychiatric illness. It was a side effect of the antipsychotic drugs she was taking. These drugs block the effect of dopamine in the brain. Dopamine plays a role in a variety of diseases. The loss of dopamine causes parkinsonism, while the increased activity of dopamine causes chorea. That is why the antipsychotic agents that block the activity of dopamine are so useful in patients with Huntington's chorea.

But blocking the activity of dopamine with antipsychotic drugs (often called neuroleptics) in turn causes akathisia. In most patients, akathisia manifests itself as a continuous motor restlessness, a need to walk continuously. In some, this compulsion may be converted to a need to dance. Or even a need to dance all night.

It is easy to imagine a plague caused not by a bacteriumlike bubonic plague or syphilis, but by a toxin, a poison that induced a state similar, if not identical to, the akathisia caused by the antipsychotic drugs. If it was a short step for Josette from pacing to dancing, the step would have been no greater in Strasbourg in 1418. And once one sufferer started to dance, it would have been natural for the others who were affected to join in. The trip to the Tomb of Saint Vitus may have cured the dancing mania because in making the trek, the sufferer finally left those areas in which the toxin was present.

What do we make of the "contagious" spread of the disease from town to town? I suspect it was more a spread of the "music," of the conversion of akathisia from pacing to dancing, than of the akathisia itself.

What was the nature of the toxin?

That is entirely speculative, but I suspect that it was a toxin produced by a fungus that infected the grain. Funguses have been shown to produce toxins that can block the activity of dopamine and would be capable of producing akathisia.

Once I made the diagnosis of akathisia, the vicious cycle of Josette's dancing mania was broken.

I put her back on a very low dose of Stelazine. That night, she listened to the radio play softly while tapping her feet. Two nights later, she slept all night.

Her akathisia was cured.

Unfortunately, I had no such cure for her Huntington's chorea.

Author's Note

The dancing mania has left us two legacies. One is a type of music, the tarantella, which was played while the afflicted danced. Somehow the belief grew that the bite of a spider, a tarantula, caused the dance, and that music cured it. This superstition became so persistent that for three hundred years tarantella players were called to cure people who were bitten by spiders. As time went on, new notions were added: the dance was supposed to bring on a perspiration that washed away the poison of the tarantula. But not quite all of it; a trace remained, so every summer the dance had to be repeated by all who had ever been bitten or thought they had or wished they had.

The story that the tarantula bite caused the dancing mania began in southern Italy and spread through the Italian peninsula. It was really just an afterthought, something to explain what the people could not understand.

The other legacy was the popularization of traveling to the shrines of various saints to seek a cure for some otherwise incurable affliction. There is a tendency to attribute any such cure to a reversal of a hysterical state. Most probably are. Are they all? I doubt if the world is such a simple place.

=17=

As Helpful as Cupping
a Corpse*

Es virt helfen vi a toytem bankes.*
    —Yiddish proverb

Nature abhors a vacuum.
    —Aristotle

'cause that's where the money is.
    —Willie Sutton

By the time I was asked to see Wallace Berger in consultation, the doctors who were treating him were almost as confused as he was. Berger was in his mid-eighties and was brought to the emergency room by one of his neighbors, who found him wandering around the backyard of their apartment building, barefoot without either a hat or coat and muttering in Yiddish. According to the neighbor, Berger normally spoke English and spoke it fairly well, albeit with a distinct accent.

Once he arrived at the emergency room, Mr. Berger lost his personal identity and became just another patient. In no time, the nurses discovered that he had a fever of 101.6 F.—not exactly a triumph of modern medicine, but it was progress. To the residents, he now became the old man with a fever. If he was admitted and turned out to be interesting, he would then

*This is a translation of the Yiddish proverb.

become "a case." Speaking Yiddish, which none of our doctors understood, was looked upon as a quaint form of behavior, but nothing to concern the ER physicians. Every day, they saw patients babbling away in
languages that none of them understood; that was part of life in a big city.
However, going outdoors in Chicago in January without a hat or coat or
even shoes when it was 3 below 0 with a wind-chill factor of minus 37 F.
was, even they recognized, truly aberrant behavior. But it wasn't their
problem. Once they figured out whether the patient had any medical disorders that needed to be treated, they could then call in one of the psychiatrists to evaluate his mental condition. It was his fever that gave them
a handle, a starting place. They were internists; they knew how to work
up a fever.

White blood count—elevated.

Differential blood count—shifted to the left.

Those were sure signs of an infection, and most likely a bacterial infection. But what was causing the fever?

They obeyed Sutton's law and started with a chest X ray—negative—
and followed with a urine analysis, which was also negative.

Having struck out on the two commonest causes of acute bacterial
infections in elderly men (pneumonia and urinary-tract infections), they
fell back on the time-honored but time-consuming process of examining
the patient. They were shocked to find that his legs were covered with
round, red, sharply demarcated areas, which were all exactly the same
size—about two inches in diameter. Those that appeared to be of more
recent origin were crowded with fresh bright red dots, suggestive of bleeding due to the rupture of small blood vessels. In others, where the bleeding
was a day or two old, the dots had coalesced, and the entire region had
become black and blue. In some of the round areas—a week old, perhaps—
the black and blue areas were streaked with yellow, while others had
turned dark red, almost violet in color.

No one had seen anything like them before, so perfectly round and all
the same size. What were they?

No one knew. Mr. Berger had become a case, a puzzle, and perhaps
even material for Grand Rounds. If they could only figure out what he
had. So they started guessing.

Kaposi's sarcoma?

From that, it was only a short jump to assume that the patient had
AIDS. What else could he have? He had Kaposi's sarcoma and an infection
of unknown cause, or FUO (fever of unknown origin, in medical slang).

They called dermatology.

The attending dermatologists had all gone home for the day; it was already 9:30 P.M. The sole dermatologist who was still around was a first-year resident, and he'd only been a dermatologist for a few months. He was also at the same disadvantage as the rest of the doctors who were caring for Mr. Berger: He was under thirty. The dermatology resident didn't think it was Kaposi's sarcoma but he didn't know what else it could be. Perhaps leprosy, he suggested.

Leprosy!

Out went a page for the infectious disease resident on call, who likewise had no idea what the skin lesions were. Of course, he'd never seen a case of leprosy. He, too, was in his first year of training and suggested it might be some sort of ring worm.

Back to the dermatology resident.

On further consideration and reference to a selection of textbooks, the dermatology resident thought it was more likely to be a rare form of vasculitis. Perhaps they should biopsy one of the skin lesions. When in doubt, do a biopsy.

But which one?

A new one or an old one?

They paged the immunology fellow to get his opinion, and then a surgeon.

And so it went. By the time I stopped by to see him the next morning, the infectious disease resident had at least managed to locate the source of Mr. Berger's fever: a skin ulcer on his left heel that had developed a small abscess. The infectious disease service had put him on antibiotics. I was asked to see him because the immunology fellow knew a little Yiddish and had been able to ask Mr. Berger a few questions. Mr. Berger thought it was 1936 and that he was running away from the Nazis, who'd caught him and thrown him into a hotel, and that the doctors were all Nazis. Technically, Mr. Berger was manifesting the altered behavior of an acute confusional state caused not by psychiatric disease but by diffuse malfunction of wide areas of the brain. He did not know where he was, what he was doing, who we were, what we were doing—or, rather, what we were *trying* to do. And he had no idea what year it was.

Several times the resident told him that it was 1984, that he was in a hospital, and that we were all doctors. Each time, he heard what he was told; each time he repeated the facts. And each time he forgot them just as quickly.

He was confused. He could neither lay down new memories nor call up most of the memories he had. But what had brought about the diffuse brain dysfunction? The list of possible causes is almost endless, and it was my job to discover the right one.

The residents wondered if the combination of psychosis and skin rash meant that Mr. Berger had a rare form of syphilis. None of them had ever seen a patient with rampant syphilis of the brain, for that disease had virtually disappeared from the American medical scene before any of them had been born.

I started by reviewing his chart. The suggestions of the various residents conjured up in my own mind possiblities of rarely seen diseases, and I, too, began to see myself as the discussant at Grand Rounds. He might even become a publishable case report. From the ER to a medical journal. I walked into his room with great expectations. The attending dermatologist was already examining the mysterious circles. He was old enough to have seen all the forms of syphilis and leprosy and just about everything else in dermatology.

The diagnostic list that the residents had conjured up during the night was formidable: Kaposi's sarcoma, vasculitis, syphilis, leprosy. None of them was a very attractive alternative.

My own list was longer and even more exotic, but no more attractive.

The dermatologist looked at me, chuckled, and said, "We biopsy a cupped man. It's better than cupping a corpse."

I knew immediately what he meant. All the arcane diagnoses that I had been hatching in my mind while reading the chart instantly disappeared. There is a long list of rare diseases that combine skin rashes and mental or neurologic problems. Some I have seen; some I've only read about. I had been hoping to make a great diagnosis of some obscure syndrome containing the name of at least two, if not three, dead physicians. But there would be no case report here, and probably no Grand Rounds, either.

Wallace Berger had no skin disease at all. The dermatologist had taken one look and had made the correct diagnosis. He was not a young doctor in training. He'd been around, and he'd seen the signs of cupping before.

In a sense, Mr. Berger didn't even have any neurologic disease. Now that his fever had cleared he was entirely rational and told us exactly what had happened. He had developed an infection on his heel. It had happened several times before, and each time he'd treated it himself. It wasn't that he didn't have confidence in doctors or trust them but . . . he believed in taking care of himself, as he always did for such minor infections. What he did was to cup himself.

He then described how he took a glass, actually an old jelly jar, and heated it, first by placing it in boiling water and then by carefully holding it over an open flame. Once it was the right temperature—and that he knew merely by the feel, for after all, he had been doing this all his life— he placed the cup, or more correctly, the jelly jar, on his leg.

He even knew why cupping worked. As the heated air within the glass cooled, it created a vacuum and pulled the skin up into the jar, since, as Mr. Berger reminded me, "Nature abhors a vacuum."

"It sucks the blood," he continued, "into the skin and pulls out the poisons."

His general concept was not that far off, but some of his details were somewhat inaccurate. Nature does not abhor a vacuum—rather, it tries to maintain equal pressures. When he heated the jar, the air within it expanded. Once the jar cooled, the gases contracted. As a result of the contraction, the pressure within the jar fell and became lower than the pressure exerted on the rest of his skin by the normal atmospheric pressure of the environment. Hence, his skin was pushed into the place of least pressure—the jelly jar. In the same way, the blood was pushed into the small capillaries of the skin. Many of these capillaries broke, causing the small red dots known as petechiae. These dots coalesced over time and changed color as the blood cells broke down.

Mr. Berger had been cupping this particular infection for about two weeks. That explained why the various cupped areas were of different colors, corresponding to their various ages.

Cupping is an old folk remedy for drawing off the bad humors. It dates back thousands of years and was once one of the mainstays of the physician's armamentarium. An Englishman, Thomas Mapleson, wrote a book in 1813 titled *A Treatise on the Art of Cupping*. At the time, Mapleson was the official cupper to His Royal Highness the Prince Regent and to Westminster Hospital and the St. Pancras Parochial Infirmary. In his book, Mapleson quoted Hippocrates on the use of cupping, and described the beneficial effect of cupping upon painful disorders, such as pleurisy and headaches, as well as throat infections. He also recommended this all but universal form of therapy in such diverse states as delerium, insanity, and "dejection of the spirits." (Our experience with Mr. Berger, whose delerium developed despite vigorous cupping, suggests that it has limited efficacy in that condition.) Mapleson believed that the earliest practitioners of the art of cupping were probably the ancient Egyptians, for cupping was then still popular in Egypt even when other treatments were more appropriate: "They are either unacquainted with the use of leeches, or have a prejudice against them."

Although cupping was often done by physicians and surgeons in the nineteenth century, it was also carried out by others whose training and skills may have been inferior. This disturbed Mapleson, who violently disapproved of advertisements for cupping at such establishments as bathhouses. These ads appeared in the popular publications of the day like *The*

Tatler and *The Spectator*. During the nineteenth century, English medicine abandoned cupping, although the technique was still described in papers from Eastern Europe as late as 1940.

Mr. Berger believed that cupping was an effective form of therapy for inflammation. Despite its apparent failure in the present situation, he was still confident that cupping usually worked. After all, he had used it many times during his life, and he was eighty-five and in pretty good shape. Lots of people he knew who scoffed at cupping had died long before they reached that age.

I couldn't deny the truth of that statement, although the syllogism that it implied was illogical.

I had been asked to see Mr. Berger because of his confusion. The confusion had cleared up as soon as his fever had gone away. But why had he been confused?

That question is one that has bothered me for all my career as a neuroscientist. The observation that fever often causes confusion, especially in older patients, is irrefutable. The mechanism behind the process remains obscure. It is probably a combination of biochemical and physiological factors. The brain differs from most other organs in that its normal function depends upon the integrated behavior of all its cells. In contrast, an organ like the liver will depend upon the additive activities of its component cells. If each liver cell is working at 80 percent capacity, the liver as a whole works at 80 percent capacity. If each brain cell works at 80 percent capacity, the brain *doesn't work*.

The function of each individual cell in the brain depends upon the ability of that cell to metabolize glucose rapidly to produce the energy needed to maintain the electrical activity of its outer membrane. The enzymes that metabolize the glucose are highly susceptible to changes in body temperature. I visualize the process in this way:

1. Fever $\rightarrow$ altered enzyme function.
2. Altered enzyme function $\rightarrow$ altered energy metabolism.
3. Altered energy metabolism $\rightarrow$ altered membrane function.
4. Altered membrane function $\rightarrow$ abnormal electrical function.
5. Abnormal electrical function $\rightarrow$ abnormal behavior.

In other words, fever $\rightarrow$ confusion. It may be more complicated than that, but that's how I imagine the process works.

Author's Note

Willie Sutton was a bank robber. His sole contribution to medicine was a quip that has become converted into a basic law. Willie never robbed anything but banks. The FBI, as well as the banks, took a dim view of such a penchant. As a result, Willie had been arrested and convicted several times, spending much of his life behind bars. When released from his last incarceration, he was interviewed by a newspaper reporter.

"Why," asked the reporter, "do you rob banks?"

" 'Cause," Willie replied, "that's where the money is."

In the day-to-day practice of medicine, Sutton's law directs physicians to go straight to the test that is most likely to give the final diagnosis, even if that test is invasive, since that procedure is "where the money is."

A patient whose symptoms were similar to those of Mr. Berger was recently published in the "Diagnosis?" section of the English journal *Lancet* by Sean Lennon and Sarah Davenport ("A Long Discontinued Practice," Lancet 2 [1987]: 1533–34.) The English physicians, who, like their young American counterparts, were all under age fifty, had great difficulty recognizing the skin lesions and making the correct diagnosis of cupping. Had I thought about it, I could have published Mr. Berger's story in a medical journal and beaten Lennon and Davenport to the punch. Berger could have become a case report. Instead, he remains just a memory and one of the stories I tell on rounds.

=18=

The Girl with Dancing Eyes

I am interested in medical research because I believe in it.
—Bernard Baruch

My adventure with the girl with dancing eyes began several years before she was born. It began in Vienna, a place that, to my knowledge, she had never visited. It began on the Ringstrasse—that circle of streets that now occupies the precise space where the walls of the old city once stood. I had first read about the Ringstrasse in a book about psychoanalysis. I was a freshman at the University of Michigan at the time and had just taken my first psychology course. More important, I was discovering classical music—not just Beethoven, Brahms, and Tschaikovsky but Stravinski, Bartók, and Mahler—especially Mahler. The book was called *Listening with the Third Ear*. It had been written by one of Freud's minor disciples, Theodor Reik, and contained innumerable asides to classical music and to the famous people Reik knew. Each page or two, another name was dropped. "When I was on the Ringstrasse with Mahler," seemed to be a major theme.

Well, here I now was on the Ringstrasse.

Not with Mahler—that would have been hoping for far too much—but with Walter Birkmayer. Birkmayer is an Austrian neurologist who by then had already come up with two of the most important clinical observations made in neurology during my professional lifetime:

1. He was one of the two neurologists who first discovered that levodopa (L-dopa) improves parkinsonism.

2. He alone demonstrated that the effect of L-dopa is increased by
   an enzyme inhibitor that alters the way in which the body metab-
   olizes L-dopa.

Together these two findings revolutionized the treatment of Parkinson's
disease. Many others subsequently made important contributions to the
development of L-dopa, but it all started with Birkmayer.

It was 1971 when I strolled along the Ringstrasse with Birkmayer. We
were discussing Parkinson's disease and its chemistry and treatment and
we were exchanging ideas and experience. And I was only three years out
of my residency.

We talked of many things. We talked about dopamine and the key role
it plays in Parkinson's disease. We talked of my animal research with
L-dopa. Birkmayer had never done much animal work, but had gone
directly from the data from human autopsies that demonstrated that Parkinson's disease was due to the loss of brain dopamine to treatment of
parkinsonian patients with L-dopa. L-dopa is the precursor of dopamine.
It can cross into the brain and once there, be converted to dopamine. This
conversion then acts to replace the dopamine lost in Parkinson's disease.

I was studying the effects of large doses of L-dopa on the behavior of
animals in the hope that these experiments would help us understand some
of the side effects that L-dopa caused in patients. I described to Birkmayer
the acute effects of L-dopa the first time an animal received it and the
chronic effects after two or three months of continuous exposure to the
drug.

Then we talked about another chemical that was reduced in the brains
of patients who died with Parkinson's disease, a chemical called serotonin.
No one knew exactly what function serotonin had in the brain, nor what
role, if any, it played in Parkinson's disease. Those same two questions
are still unanswered today.

Birkmayer asked whether I had ever studied serotonin.

No I hadn't, but I knew that a small molecule known as
5-hydroxytryptophan, or 5-HTP, was the precursor of serotonin and could
enter the brain and become converted to serotonin in the same way that
L-dopa is converted to dopamine—and by the very same enzyme.

Had I ever given 5-HTP to any guinea pigs? Birkmayer questioned.

No, I hadn't.

Later that night, I called Chicago to talk to one of the medical students
who was working in my laboratory. This student had been interested in
finding a simple project that she could do on her own, and when I had left
for Vienna, I hadn't yet come up with one, but promised her I would

continue to think about it. Well, now I had the idea, Birkmayer's idea. I told her to give 5-HTP to guinea pigs to see what would happen.

"What *will* happen?" she asked.

"I have no idea," I replied.

"Then why?"

"To see what will happen. It's called research."

"Why guinea pigs? Why not rats? Rats are less expensive."

"Two reasons," I explained. We knew more about the chemistry of the guinea pig and much more about its normal behavior. "Besides, I hate rats," I added.

It took about twenty minutes more for me to outline the various experiments that had to be set up, and by the time I was done, she, too, was interested in the project.

After Vienna, I traveled to Israel for a much-needed vacation, and returned to Chicago, my patients, and my laboratory about a month later.

Actually, I didn't have time to visit the lab until I had been back at the hospital for several days and had caught up with my clinical work. When I did make it to the laboratory, the woman whom I had talked to from Vienna collared me immediately.

"They bounce," she said.

"Who?"

"The guinea pigs; they bounce like kernels of popcorn."

This I had to see.

I watched as she injected some normal guinea pigs with 5-HTP. For the first five minutes, nothing happened. The earliest abnormal behavior that I saw was a form of exaggerated grooming behavior. The animals appeared to brush their faces and scratch their sides with their paws, at first intermittently and then all but continuously. Just when the grooming behavior peaked, the second behavioral alteration began: a sudden shaking or jerking of the head and neck. These jerks were also initially intermittent, but they quickly became continuous and almost rhythmic. Then the most impressive behavioral manifestation started: a peculiar rhythmic bouncing of the animals that evolved from the head and neck tremor. The animals appeared to jump straight up from the floor of the cage, often propelled forward or backward. Not infrequently, the guinea pigs had all four feet off the floor at the same time.

I was impressed. Did all the animals bounce?

That depended on the dose of 5-HTP they had been given. At 100 mg., none bounced; at 200 mg., one out of four bounced; and at 300 mg., they all bounced.

The frequency of the bouncing was also dose related: At 300 mg., the guinea pigs bounced at a rate of 60 bounces per minute; at 400 mg., they bounced at a rate of 80 to 100 bounces per minute.

"What should we do next?" the student asked.

"We'll measure the effect of 5-HTP on brain serotonin levels and see if the bouncing correlates with elevation in brain serotonin."

"Anything else?"

"Don't give it to any elephants."

Two weeks later at our weekly laboratory meeting the student presented the results. 5-HTP did increase brain serotonin, which we expected, since it was the precursor of serotonin. More important, the degree of serotonin increase was related to the severity of the bouncing behavior.

So we now had a way of observing and quantifying one effect of serotonin in the brain of a healthy animal and we knew one thing that serotonin did: It caused bouncing, whatever that meant.

An animal model of popcorn, she suggested.

Her reply was not as sarcastic as it sounds. My laboratory spent most of its efforts in those years studying animal behaviors as models or analogies of human diseases. Here we had a behavior without a disease, a model without a home. Like a cure without an illness, it was not much good to anyone.

I was the clinician, the specialist in human behaviors, normal and abnormal. It was my job to find the human analogy.

"By the way," the medical student added, "I'm not afraid to give 5-HTP to an elephant. It would be interesting."

"You're not?" The vision of an elephant bouncing up and down with all four limbs off the ground at once struck fear into my heart. God knows what would happen. "You're a braver man than I, Gunga Din," I said.

"I don't know about that. But I've given 5-HTP to rats and mice and cats."

"What happened?"

"Very little. And none of them bounced."

She spent the next few months trying to figure out why the guinea pigs bounced but the rats didn't. I spent the next two years trying to figure out what the bouncing meant, if anything.

I once walked into the laboratory just as the injected guinea pigs were at the height of their grooming behavior, before they had commenced the head jerks or bouncing. I dropped a heavy medical book on the table next to the observation cage, and it slapped down with a sharp thud.

The pigs bounced, all six of them, one single bounce each, and all six at the same time.

I lifted up the book again and dropped it.

Thud.

All six guinea pigs bounced up off the floor of the cage.

Each time I dropped the book, a sudden bounce followed.

"Stimulus-sensitive bouncing," I said.

"So?" came the response from my student.

"It's a perfect animal model of the jumping Frenchmen of Maine."

"Of what?" she asked.

I tried to explain. The "jumping Frenchmen of Maine" was the name given to a neurologic disorder that had been described in some French trappers who lived in Maine in the 1880s. Sudden noises caused them to jump.

Had I ever seen such a patient? No.

Had anyone I ever knew seen one? No.

She thought I should keep looking for my human analogy. A model of a disease no one had seen since the nineteenth century was unlikely to change the course of American neurology.

The medical student finished her six-month stint in our lab, graduated from medical school, and went on to take her residency in psychiatry. The lab became more deeply involved with other projects, and no one had time to watch guinea pigs bounce.

It was two years later that I first saw Debra Marshall. She was just under two years old and had been perfectly well until about a month before. She was the Marshalls's first child. Her father, Willard, was 36 and in good health and had no familial diseases. Her mother, Phyllis, was 28; also in good health; and, as far as she knew, her family had no neurologic problems.

The pregnancy had been normal—Phyllis had no illnesses and had taken no medicine—and was followed by a normal delivery.

Debra had started walking by age one and by the time she was a year and a half, she was using short sentences.

Then, a month ago, her head began to twitch. The twitches occurred only rarely at first, once every five or ten minutes, but then grew more frequent and more powerful, until they were not just twitches, but real jerks that all but knocked her over.

Now they were almost continuous, and it was not just her head that jerked, but her entire body. She no longer walked, since the jerks knocked her down, so she was forced to crawl. Even then, her jerks caused problems, sometimes they were so severe that they lifted her off the ground like a piece of popcorn.

Popcorn!

And when she lay in bed, her legs kept on moving regularly, as if she were dancing to some unheard song. So did her eyes.

She had dancing eyes and dancing legs. I had read that description before. *Dancing eyes and dancing legs.*

Phyllis brought Debra into one of my examining rooms and laid her on her back.

Debra's eyes were dancing. They moved continuously, not in any regular pattern that I could discern, but irregularly—chaotically, in fact, in all directions, at different rates.

Her arms jerked, and her legs as well, but even more dramatically, as if she were doing a complex dance, choreographed by a choreographer gone berserk.

There was one more symptom to check: I had to see her bounce like a piece of popcorn.

Carefully, I lifted her and put her into a crawling position, so that she supported herself on her hands and knees.

Debra was frightened and began to cry softly. Something bad was going to happen to her.

When nothing happened, I clapped my hands as loudly as I could—a single loud crack.

She jerked.

Her head tossed back.

Her arms and legs thrust down, and she bounced up, all four of her limbs lifting off the table simultaneously.

She had bounced up like a piece of popcorn.

Her mother screamed.

Debra fell back on the table, crying.

I smiled—triumph. I knew what her bouncing meant, and the bouncing of my guinea pigs, as well. My animal model was no longer an orphan. More important than that, I had an idea as to what was happening to little Debra, or at least I thought I did, and I suspected there was a chance that she could be cured. I'd never seen a patient with dancing eyes and dancing feet before, but I'd seen my own bouncing guinea pigs, and they all had normal brains. It was just possible that Debra also had a normal brain.

The Marshalls were as frightened as their daughter. They had seen one neurologist and several pediatricians. None of them had given them any hope. These doctors all thought that Debra had a progressive disease of the brain, and the Marshalls could only believe them. After all, they had watched the jerks get worse and worse.

Could anything be done to help Debra?

To make her more comfortable?

I thought so, and even thought she might have something we might be able to cure.

What?

A tumor, I said.

A brain tumor? they asked.

No. To me the nature of her bouncing suggested that her brain was normal.

Why?

I told them about my guinea pigs.

They were far from convinced. What about her other movements?

According to what I recalled, the syndrome of dancing eyes and dancing feet had been described in two separate conditions in young children. Some of the children had inflammation of the base of the brain, a condition called brain stem encephalitis. Others had a tumor, not of the brain, but somewhere else in the body, usually in the chest. And these tumors, called neuroblastomas, were usually benign. If Debra had a neuroblastoma, and if the neuroblastoma was benign, then we could cure her. Because of her popcornlike jumps, I was betting on the neuroblastoma.

I admitted Debra to the hospital.

Her chest X ray showed a tumor, and further evaluation revealed no evidence of malignant spread.

Two days later, the surgeons operated on Debra.

The tumor was a neuroblastoma, a benign neuroblastoma. The surgeons removed it totally.

The next morning her eyes were no longer dancing. Nor were her feet. Within three days, she was crawling, and even the loudest noise had no effect on her. She went home ten days afterward, a normal two year old.

Her tumor never returned, nor did the dancing eyes or dancing feet, nor her stimulus-sensitive bouncing.

I called the ex-medical student who had done all the initial work on 5-HTP in my lab and told her all about Debra Marshall.

She understood immediately. Stimulus-sensitive bouncing had been the normal response of the intact brain of normal guinea pigs given 5-HTP. Debra had stimulus-sensitive bouncing. Her brain, like those of the guinea pigs, was normal, but some chemical much like 5-HTP had to have been acting on her brain. That chemical had to have come from the neuroblastoma.

Our animal model was no longer in search of a disease.

When I finally wrote up our work on 5-HTP-induced bouncing in guinea pigs as an animal model of stimulus-sensitive myoclonus (bouncing) in children, it sounded much more logical, almost as if the clinical setting had led to subsequent animal studies. The last paragraph of this article summarized what we knew at that time:

> The clinical setting that implicates humoral mechanisms in the production of myoclonic movements is the occurrence of these movements in infants with neuroblastomas. These tumors produce a wide variety of active chemicals. The occasional rapid improvement in patients with these movements after removal of the tumor supports the concept that the tumor is producing a substance that crosses the blood-brain barrier and produces the movement abnormality. Evidence exists that 5-HTP or other serotonin-related precursors may be produced by these tumors. A single case of a 56-year-old man with neuroblastoma has been reported in which there was excretion of 5-HTP in the urine. This case shows that neuroblastomas can produce 5-HTP and suggests that patients presenting with dancing eyes, dancing feet and stimulus-sensitive myoclonus had a normal nervous system responding in a normal way to excessive chemical stimulation with 5-HTP.

Whenever I hear Mahler now, I remember the Ringstrasse and Walter Birkmayer and Debra Marshall.

It's not a bad memory.

Author's Note

Our original work with bouncing guinea pigs is H. L. Klawans, C. G. Goetz, and W. J. Weiner, "5-Hydroxytryptophan Induced Myoclonus in Guinea Pigs and the Possible Role of Serotonin in Infantile Myoclonus." *Neurology* (1973) 23:1234–40.

The three most important clinical reports on which my diagnosis of Debra Marshall was based were these:

1. M. Kinsbourne, "Myocloic Encephaolopathy of Infants," *Journal of Neurology, Neurosurgery and Psychiatry* 25 (1962): 271–76.

2. P. Dyken and O. Kolar, "Dancing Eyes, Dancing Feet: Infantile Polymyoclonia," *Brain* 91 (1968): 305–19.

3. P. G. Moe and G. Nellhaus, "Infantile Polymyocloniaopsoclonus Syndrome and Neural Crest Tumors." *Neurology* (Minneapolis) 20 (1970): 756–64.

Shortly after my article appeared, I received another phone call from the woman who had worked on 5-HTP in my lab.

"I'm glad I didn't give any 5-HTP to an elephant," she said.

"Why?"

"Some researchers from the psychiatry department at UCLA did some studies on elephants," she explained.

"You've got to be kidding."

"They gave an elephant LSD."

"Why?"

"To see what happened."

"What happened?"

"The elephant died."

There didn't seem to be a reasonable answer.

=19=

Getting a Kick from Cocaine

Some get a kick from cocaine.
I'm sure that if
I took even one sniff,
it would bore me terrifically too.
> —Cole Porter, "I Get a Kick Out of You"

Quick, Watson, the needle.
> —Sherlock Holmes in the movie *The Hound of the Baskervilles,*
> starring Basil Rathbone and Nigel Bruce

John H. Watson, MD:
The most famous and best beloved physician in literature.
> —Vincent Starrett, author of the first biography of Sherlock Holmes

On May 4, 1891, Mr. Sherlock Holmes, the first and still the most well known of the world's ever-expanding list of consulting detectives, disappeared, apparently having fallen into the chasm below Reichenbach Falls in a final life-and-death struggle with Professor Moriarty, the infamous Napoleon of crime who had long been his chief adversary. In his chronicle of the adventure, "The Final Problem," Dr. John H. Watson, who had hurried back to the top of the falls only to find a farewell note from Holmes, described the scene as follows:

A few words may suffice to tell the little that remains. An examination by experts leaves little doubt that a personal contest between the two men ended, as it could hardly fail to end in such a situation, in their reeling over, locked in each other's arms. Any attempt at recovering the bodies was absolutely hopeless, and there, deep down in that dreadful cauldron of swerling water and seething foam, will lie for all time the most dangerous criminal and the foremost champion of the law of their generation.

Almost three years later, on April 5, 1894, Holmes suddenly and unexpectedly reappeared in London. Where had he been during those three missing years? Why had he remained away so long? According to Holmes, he stayed underground to avoid the dangerous remnants of Professor Moriarty's organization, returning to his old rooms at 221 B Baker Street to dispose of Colonel Sebastian Moran, the last surviving henchman of Moriarty. This story was recorded by Watson as "The Adventure of the Empty House." Holmes offered Watson the following explanation of his whereabouts during his long absence:

I travelled for two years in Tibet, therefore, and amused myself by visiting Lhassa and spending some days with the head Llama. You may have read of the remarkable explorations of a Norwegian named Sigerson, but I am sure that it never occurred to you that you were receiving news of your friend. I then passed through Persia, looked in at Mecca, and paid a short but interesting visit to the Khalifa at Khartoum, the results of which I have communicated to the Foreign Office. Returning to France I spent some months in a research into the coal-tar derivatives, which I conducted in a laboratory at Montpelier, in the South of France. Having concluded this to my satisfaction, and learning that only one of my enemies was now left in London, I was about to return when my movements were hastened by the news of this remarkable Park Lane Mystery, which not only appealed to me by its own merits, but which seemed to offer some most peculiar personal opportunities.

In a 1968 article published in the *Journal of the American Medical Association,* Dr. David Musto offered an alternative explanation. He proposed that for much of the three years, Holmes was in Vienna, living in the home of Dr. Sigmund Freud and being treated by Freud for his cocaine addiction. The same hypothesis was expanded by Nicholas Meyer in *The Seven Percent Solution.* Meyer's 1971 novel claims to be based on detailed notes of John H. Watson, MD, which could not be revealed during Holmes's lifetime. Because of the supposed authenticity of this source, the Musto-Meyer hypothesis is now considered to reflect what actually transpired during the missing three years in the life of Sherlock Holmes.

To accept this theory, the reader of Watson's chronicles of the life and adventures of Holmes is asked to believe that Holmes, the possessor of that "admirably balanced mind," was a victim of cocaine addiction and that he had traveled all the way to Vienna to seek the help of Sigmund Freud, who in 1891 was a rather obscure neurologist. Holmes's visit, in fact, was supposed to have occured several years before Freud had published his first major psychiatric work: Josef Breuer and Freud's pivotal *Studies on Hysteria,* which was Freud's first published book in psychiatry, did not appear in print until 1895, four years after Holmes's disappearance. If Freud had any international reputation at the time of Holmes's visit, it was for his work in pediatric neurology, and for his having translated the lectures of the great French neurologist Jean Marie Charcot from French into German. This was no minor feat. Charcot (see Chapter 7, "The Man About Town"), was then the leading neurologist in the world. The first professor of neurology in the world. Freud, like many others, had traveled to Paris to spend some time studying with him. Freud's translation, however, would have produced little, if any, renown in English-speaking countries, where physicians were more likely to read Charcot in the original French than in a German translation.

All in all, the cocaine-Freud hypothesis seems to raise more questions than it answers. Was Holmes really a cocaine addict? How could Holmes, who rarely left London, much less England, have heard of Sigmund Freud? And, more precisely, how could Holmes have known that Freud was aware of the dangers of cocaine addiction, let alone that he was even trying to cure such patients? This hypothesis becomes even more of a problem when one considers that Freud had written a series of medical papers (in German), all of which had proclaimed the wonders of cocaine and had vehemently discounted any possibility that cocaine itself had any addicting or dangerous properties.

Cocaine is derived from two closely related species of shrubs that are native to South America. Bolivian coca comes from the Andes highland forests, although a closely related variety grows in the Amazon lowland basin. Colombian coca grows in Colombia and Venezuela and on the desert coast of Peru. By the time Europeans first reached South America, the use of coca, the source of cocaine, had already become widespread there. Manco Capac, the royal son of the Sun God, was believed to have given coca directly to the Incas. In turn, the Inca priests had declared that coca itself was divine. In the Inca culture, coca was chewed in a mixture called *cocada,* which was made up of coca, an alkali that would act to release the active ingredients from the coca leaves, and some sort of binding material. The importance of coca to the pre-Columbian culture is reflected by the fact that the term *cocada* came to be used as a measure of distance—the distance a man could walk under the influence of cocaine—or of time—40 minutes, or the duration of the action of cocaine when taken orally.

The first description of the peculiar effects of coca to reach Europe was written in the sixteenth century by Nicolás Monardes of Spain, but for some reason the plant aroused little, if any, interest until the middle of the nineteenth century. Even the description written by the early seventeenth-century chronicler of the Incas Garcilaso de la Vega—"coca satisfies the hungry, gives new strength to the weary and exhausted and makes the unhappy forget their sorrows"—did nothing to "turn on" seventeenth-century Europeans. Most Europeans were far more interested in another plant that Monardes described in the same book—tobacco.

This was not the case, however, in the middle of the nineteenth century. In 1859, an Italian physician, Paolo Montegazza, published a pamphlet based on his own experiences during his travels among Peruvian Indians and proclaimed that coca was a wonderous new weapon against various diseases. Unlike the little-heralded work of Monardes, Montegazza's report attracted a great deal of attention. The following year, Alfred Niemann, a Viennese biochemist, succeeded in purifying coca alkaloid and named it cocaine. The first scientific reports on the effects of cocaine were relatively unenthusiastic, but, of course, quality control in the use of coca leaves and its extracts was poor at best.

While the scientific community was slow to study cocaine, the public was quick to adapt its use. In 1865, "Vin Mariani," a preparation of wine and coca leaves, was placed on the European market. By 1890, a wide variety of cocaine nostrums were being sold, including cocaine cordials and even coca cigarettes. The foremost of these was Coca-Cola, which contained true "coke" when it was first concocted. The popular press in Europe and America carried numerous articles proclaiming the wonders of cocaine. Holmes was, as is well known from the various descriptions by Watson, a voracious reader of the popular press and so must have been well aware of the potential benefits of cocaine.

But was Holmes a cocaine addict? The unequivocal answer is yes. In "A Scandal in Bohemia" (probably late 1886), Watson tells us that Holmes "who loathes every form of society with his whole Bohemian soul, remained in our lodgings in Baker Street, buried among his old books, and alternating from week to week between cocaine and ambition, the drowsiness of the drug, and the fierce energy of his own keen nature." Watson had seen little of Holmes because of Watson's recent marriage. He called upon Holmes at their old lodging and noted that Holmes had "risen out of his drug-created dreams and was hot upon the scent of some new problem."

The next year, in "The Man With the Twisted Lip," Watson worries that Holmes's drug habits may be increasing and receives the following tart reply from the detective: "I suppose, Watson," said he, "that you imagine that I have added opium smoking to cocaine injections, and all the other weaknesses on which you have favored me with your medical views." But no, Holmes was in the opium den in pursuit of a criminal, not his own pleasure.

A few months later, in "the Five Orange Pips," Watson referred to Holmes as a "self poisoner by cocaine and tobacco."

In 1888, Watson reported, "Save for the occasional use of cocaine, he had no vices, and he only turned to the drug as a protest against the monotony of existence when cases were scanty and the papers uninteresting" (The Yellow Face). The longest discussion of the detective's cocaine habit appears that same year in The Sign of the Four:

> Sherlock Holmes took his bottle from the corner of the mantelpiece, and his hypodermic syringe from its neat morocco case. With his long, white, nervous fingers he adjusted the delicate needle and rolled back his left shirt-cuff. For some little time his eyes rested thoughtfully upon the sinewy fore-arm and wrist, all dotted and scarred with innumerable puncture-marks. Finally, he thrust the sharp home, pressed down the tiny piston, and sank back into the velvet-lined armchair with a long sigh of satisfaction.
>
> Three times a day for many months I had witnessed this performance, but custom had not reconciled my mind to it. . . .
>
> "Which is it to-day," I asked, "morphine or cocaine?"
>
> He raised his eyes languidly from the old black-letter volume which he had opened.
>
> "It is cocaine," he said, "a seven-per-cent solution. Would you care to try it?"
>
> "No indeed," I answered brusquely. "My constitution has not got over the Afghan campaign yet. I cannot afford to throw any extra strain upon it."

The various stories recorded by Dr. John Watson make it all too clear that Holmes was a confirmed cocaine addict long before the missing period of his life (1891–94). Was he still addicted after these three years had passed? A careful study of all Watson's many writings reveals that there is no reference to cocaine abuse by Holmes in any stories dated later than 1894, when Holmes returned to London. In The Adventure of the Missing

Three-quarter, which took place in 1896, Watson remarks that Holmes had been weaned of his drug mania, but the good doctor still worried that a period of idleness could rekindle Holmes's craving for an artificial stimulus. All in all, the historical evidence strongly points not only to Holmes being a cocaine addict, but to the conclusion that he overcame his addiction sometime between 1891 and 1894.

Did his addiction affect Holmes's behavior? Or was it merely a "recreational drug" that he used to relieve his boredom?

The records of his friend John H. Watson once again supply the necessary clinical details. Holmes clearly developed what we would today diagnose as a cocaine-induced psychosis. Most commonly, such psychoses are characterized by grandiose and paranoid thoughts, as well as a tangential grasp of reality. In "The Final Problem," all these elements come out in his conversations with Watson:

> "You have probably never heard of Professor Moriarity?" said he.
> "Never."
> "Ay, there's the genius and the wonder of the thing!" he cried. "The man pervades London and no one has heard of him. That's what puts him on a pinnacle in the records of crime."

Similar evidence abounds in this and other stories dating from around 1891. No such evidence can be found after 1894.

By the 1880s, the abuse of cocaine was widespread in both Europe and the United States. The first published reports of the medical use of coca or its alkaloid derivatives appeared in American medical periodicals. In 1876, writing in the then-prestigious *Boston Medical and Surgical Journal,* Dr. G. A. Stockwell described numerous possible therapeutic benefits from coca, provided, of course, that it was not used in excess. Stockwell proclaimed that coca eliminated fatigue without causing depression and that there was "no recoil" from this use of the agent. He concluded that "the moderate use of coca is not only wholesome but frequently beneficial." Stockwell believed that only alarmists could be worried about any possible habituation.

Four years later, several articles in the *Therapeutic Gazette* suggested that coca was a "new cure for the opium habit"; that coca could be used by addicts in place of opium; and that after it had replaced opium, coca could be easily and safely withdrawn, leaving the one-time addict free of addiction. The first of these brief reports, written by Edward D. Huse,

suggested that coca cured only the opium habit, while W. H. Bentley and
A. F. Stimmel, in separate papers, claimed that coca cured both alcoholism
and opium addiction. Dr. Bentley further stated that coca cured a variety
of other chronic diseases, ranging from dyspepsia to tuberculosis. It would
be presumptuous to suggest that the grandiosity of these claims raises the
possibility that it was not only the patients who had ingested coca. Be that
as it may, some of the medical literature was filled with numerous other
reports from America that were equally enthusiastic.

Sigmund Freud's original interest in cocaine was the direct result of the
suggestion that cocaine might have a specific therapeutic use in the treatment of addiction. But why was Freud so particularly drawn to this issue?
It was a far cry from his major concerns at the time—cerebral palsy and
disorders of speech. Freud's interest in cocaine was stimulated specifically
by these articles, as it happened, because Freud himself was frantically
searching for a cure for morphine addiction.

By 1883, Freud had become a close friend of another young medical
scientist, Ernst von Fleischl, who was working in Vienna. This friendship
had begun when they were studying together at the University of Vienna.
Fleischl, a brilliant physiologist, apparently developed severe, chronic pain
in his thumb following an accidental injury. It is said that he had turned
to morphine for relief from this pain and had quickly become a morphine
addict. Whatever the exact circumstances of his acquiring the morphine
habit, there is no question that Fleischl was addicted. Freud, intrigued by
what he had read in the American literature, obtained a shipment of cocaine from Eli Merck in the United States in the hope that he could use it
to cure his friend and colleague.

After several months of administering cocaine to Fleischl and taking it
himself, Freud wrote the first of his five articles on coca. This article,
entitled "Über Coca," or "About Coca," was a glowing report that suggested seven successful therapeutic applications for coca:

1. To increase the physical capacity of the body for a short time,
   which might be valuable in wartime
2. To alleviate digestive disorders of the stomach
3. To treat cachexia
4. To counteract the morphine withdrawal syndrome
5. To treat asthma
6. To stimulate sexual desire (an aphrodisiac)
7. To be used as a local anesthetic

Freud did not claim to have discovered all these uses and clearly credited
Bentley with being the first to demonstrate the value of cocaine for the

treatment of both morphine addiction and alcoholism. Freud did not merely repeat Bentley's original claims, however; he extended them and proclaimed that cocaine was so potent and specific in both morphine and alcohol addiction that with its use, alcohol asylums could soon be eliminated.

It would have been obvious to any active reader of the medical literature that Freud knew and loved cocaine. He proclaimed its virtues early and often, and his interest in it was widely known. In print, Freud always maintained that cocaine was a wonder drug and that, by itself, it was not addicting.

Unfortunately for both Freud and Fleischl, cocaine was no more successful as a cure for morphine addiction than was heroin, which had also been originally introduced in European medicine for that purpose. Furthermore, reports that suggested that cocaine was addicting began to appear in medical publications, such as the prestigious and widely read English journal, *The Lancet:*

To The Editors of The Lancet

Sirs,—I have a patient who suffers from cocaine craving. I find it impossible to keep cocaine out of his reach. This habit has brought him into a very low state of health. Perhaps some of your readers might be able to give me some suggestion as to treatment. I have tried the usual remedies in vain. He suffers from great nervousness, sleeplessness, and has become very thin.— I am, Sirs, yours truly,
Oct. 28th, 1890   Irene

Today, it is well accepted that the chronic use of cocaine fosters progressive behavioral change, and by so doing eventually causes a true psychosis. Although Freud could not have anticipated such discoveries, he did know something about the dangers of the drug. He had seen what it had done to his friend Fleischl, who under Freud's care had become addicted to cocaine. He was attempting to find some way to wean his friend from his addiction to cocaine.

Freud's papers on cocaine caused great controversy and ultimately outright rebuke from the scientific establishment. The great Viennese scientist Richard Erlenmeyer carried out his own careful study of the use of cocaine in morphine addictions and denounced it. More than just attacking cocaine, however, Erlenmeyer denounced Freud for propagating what he called the "Third Scourge of Mankind" (alcohol and morphine being the first two). Although Freud never accepted Erlenmeyer's conclusions, he withdrew his open support for cocaine as a cure for morphine addiction. He did not do so with public admission that cocaine was capable of causing addiction, but because he believed that the personalities of addicts were such that they transferred their tendency to be addicted from one drug to another. He was convinced that such individuals were so weak in will power and so susceptible that cocaine merely replaced morphine. Freud continued to hold that cocaine was not addicting, stating in his fifth and final paper on cocaine that "cocaine has claimed no victim who has not previously been addicted to another drug."

That report was published in 1887, a short three years after the enthusiastic, if not proselytizing, "Über Coca." This paper ended his rather brief professional involvement with the drug. What began with a bang, ended in a whisper, if not a whimper. In future years, Freud rarely, if ever, publicly discussed this cocaine interlude. In analytic terms, the entire adventure had resulted in a narcissistic injury that he consciously tried to suppress.

With this public stance, then, how would Sherlock Holmes or his medical amanuensis have known that Freud recognized the danger of cocaine addiction and was actually treating patients for it? Nicholas Meyer, in *The Seven Percent Solution,* would have us believe that Dr. Stamford, an obscure pathologist whose only credential was that he originally introduced Watson and Holmes, knew about Freud's work in treating cocaine addiction. How Stamford, quietly pursuing pathology in the basement of St. Bartholomew's Hospital in London, would be aware of these unpublished interests of a not well-known Viennese neurologist has never been explained. The works of Freud's that Stamford could have read had denied that cocaine was addicting.

Only someone who was acquainted with Freud or had connections in Vienna who knew him personally, could possibly have been privy to Freud's real feelings about cocaine. The fact that Irene Adler, the only woman ever to fascinate Sherlock Holmes ["that woman"], was a citizen of the Austro-Hungarian Empire raises the possibility that some member of her family in Vienna may have personally known Sigmund Freud. Perhaps her cousin, Alfred Adler, one of Freud's greatest students, may have been the missing link? Unfortunately, Freud's experience with cocaine antedates his interest in psychoanalysis by many years, and Adler was not to become his protogé until ten years after Holmes returned to London.

David Musto suggested that the note in *Lancet* signed Irene was from Watson (using the name of "that woman"—Irene Adler) and that a reply to this query may have supplied Watson with the information he needed. But the answer could come only from someone who knew Freud closely and knew his innermost feelings. Who could that have been?

As always, the best way to solve a problem involving Sherlock Holmes is to study the stories told by John Watson, MD, and recorded by Arthur Conan Doyle, MD. In "The Adventure of the Empty House," Holmes himself supplied the solution: "You may have read of the remarkable explorations of a Norwegian named Sigerson, but I am sure it never occurred to you that you were receiving news of your friend."

The name "Sigerson," the name chosen by Holmes to cover his missing three years, is the necessary clue. It ws Sigerson who had sent Holmes to Freud and made it possible for Freud to free Holmes of his cocaine addiction.

But who was Sigerson?

He was not a Norwegian explorer, but a neurologist. His full name was George Sigerson, and he was a man of great accomplishments, as demonstrated in his published list of honors: licentiate of the King and Queen's College of Physicians of Ireland and dean of the college's Faculty of Science; member of the Royal Irish Academy; fellow of the Linnean Society of London; member of the Council of the Statistical Society, Dublin; member of the Scientific Society of Brussels; and corresponding member of the Clinical and Anthropological Societies of Paris; among others.

But was Sigerson in a position to knew Freud's true feelings about cocaine and cocaine addiction?

Sigerson, like Freud, had attended Charcot's lectures at the Salpetrière and was, like Freud, a student of the father of French neurology. Although it was Freud who translated Charcot's *Lectures on the Diseases of the Nervous System* into German, it was Sigerson who translated these same lectures into English. Like many other students who find themselves coming together to study under the same master, a bond had been established between Freud and Sigerson. As a result of this bond, Sigerson was probably the only person in Great Britain who was in a position to have knowledge of Freud's private opinions as to the dangers of cocaine and Freud's interest in treating cocaine addicts. Therefore, it must have been Sigerson who answered the plea signed "Irene" and who was thereby instrumental in introducing Holmes to Freud. Holmes's use of the name "Sigerson" is his public expression of thanks to the physician who made it possible for him to spend some time with the head lama of psychoanalysis. Whether Holmes influenced the development of Freud's thinking, as Musto suggested, Freud obviously influenced Holmes's thinking and made it possible for him to become active once again as the world's foremost consulting detective, and for that we must all be thankful.

Author's Note

All the dates relating to the life of Sherlock Holmes are from the chronological data assembled by William S. Baring-Gould. Further details of this chronology can be found in two publications:

1. W. S. Baring-Gould, *Sherlock Holmes of Baker Street: A Life of the World's First Consulting Detective* (New York: Bramball House, 1962).

2. W. S. Baring-Gould, *The Annotated Sherlock Holmes* (New York: Potter, 1967). All quotations from the original stories are from this source.

Vincent Starrett's biography of Holmes *The Private Life of Sherlock Holmes* has appeared in two editions (New York: Macmillan, 1933; Chicago: University of Chicago Press, 1960); the latter is a revised and enlarged version of the former.

The notion that Sherlock Holmes was a cocaine addict is self-evident from the works of John Watson, MD, but another physician, David Musto, must be given full credit for first demonstrating the Viennese connection (*Journal of the American Medical Association:* 204 [1968]: 125–30). Sigmund Freud's adventures with cocaine are documented in Robert Buck, ed., *Cocaine Papers of Sigmund Freud* (New York: Stonehill, 1974), but the entire episode is not well covered in the standard psychoanalytically oriented biographies written by the various disciples of Freud, and Freud never publicly retracted his broad endorsement of cocaine.

I have worked on this essay in various forms for several years. An earlier version, aimed at a professional audience, appeared in *The Medicine of History,* (New York: Raven Press, 1982). A friend of mine, playwright Susan Lieberman, while editing a previous version, realized that she did not know whether Sherlock Holmes had lived or not. She took a random poll of people who worked with her at the Chicago Mercantile Exchange. They were divided 50–50 on the issue. She finally realized that her question could not be answered by a democratic process, so she called me for final confirmation. "It is," I said, "a matter of faith. Like the existence of Moses, although there is less evidence to support the latter."

=20=

Morbid Obesity

You can't be either too rich or too thin.
—Dorothy Parker

MORBID OBESITY.

The words themselves disgust. The world may love a fat man, but certainly not one who is morbidly obese. I'm not certain when that official diagnostic term came into existence. When I was in medical school, we were taught to call fat patients fat or, if we felt literate, obese. By the time I finished my neurology training, however, internists and surgeons were using the phrase "morbid obesity."

Patricia Seerey was morbidly obese, and she knew it. She'd been fat for most of her life and by the time she was in high school, she had reached her present state. Her body weight was more than twice her ideal weight. Diets came and diets went; she'd tried them all—rice, grapefruit, Pritikin, Weight Watchers—but nothing helped. She'd been through diet pills and hypnosis. Her girth remained unchanged. There seemed to be only two alternatives—staying obese or undergoing a surgical procedure, such as the removal of part of her stomach (a partial gastric resection). This operation would greatly curtail the amount of food the stomach could hold and thereby limit the amount she could eat. She hated being obese even more than she hated the idea of surgery, so she underwent the surgery. That was two years before she and I crossed paths.

Our first interaction did not involve her directly. It was late on a Tuesday afternoon. I had seen all my patients for the day and was trying to begin work on a paper based on some research we had just completed in my laboratory when my direct line rang. The call was from a lawyer, a good friend of mine. Jeff represented plaintiffs in malpractice suits and had consulted with me on several cases in the past.

Jeff told me all about Pat Seerey. She had been thirty-two years old when disaster struck. She'd always been a heavy girl.

"How heavy?" I asked.

"Very heavy."

"Morbid obesity," I suggested, just to prove that I knew the latest terminology.

"Yes, and she'd tried everything. Nothing worked. So she was referred to a surgeon, Jack Onslow."

The name meant nothing to me.

According to Jeff, Onslow was a general surgeon who frequently performed operations on patients with morbid obesity.

Pat was 5 feet 6 inches and had weighed 363 pounds. That was morbid enough for Onslow, and he admitted her to the hospital for surgery.

"What procedure?" I asked.

"A gastric resection."

That meant that he had removed most of Pat's stomach. As a result she would no longer be able to eat very much, and, consequently, would lose weight. She might never get down as far as pleasingly plump, but she might lose enough to drop the "morbid" and become full figured.

The operation went well; no complications were recorded. She was discharged from the hospital in eight days and went home.

Then the problems began. She started vomiting.

Some vomiting is common after that procedure. The new, smaller stomach is easily overstretched, and food tends to force its way back up into the esophagus. To avoid vomiting, the patient has to eat less, which most patients get used to in a short time.

"How often?" I asked.

Every day, I was told. Several times per day. In fact, whenever she ate. Especially after she ate any protein.

She started to eat less. Afterall, she was not ineducable.

"Did the vomiting persist?"

"Yes."

She started to lose weight.

"How much?"

"Ninety pounds."

"In how long?"

"In less than three months."

And the vomiting never stopped.

She came back to the hospital once to have a thorough evaluation (a *workup,* in medical terminology) to see if anything other than over filling her small stomach might be causing her vomiting. Neither Onslow nor Lyons, her internist, could find anything else wrong with her.

The vomiting continued, as did the weight loss, and she was soon down to 231 pounds. She'd lost over 130 pounds, and a full figure wasn't far off. No more muumuus for her.

But then she began to notice a burning sensation in her feet. At first it was very mild, but in a few days, her feet were burning severely from morning to night.

She went to see Onslow, who sent her to Lyons. After all, Onslow was just her surgeon and didn't know anything about burning feet.

Lyons, in turn, sent her to Frank Baker, a neurologist. Baker thought she might have a mild neuritis—inflammation of the nerves of her legs and feet. He ordered an EMG and explained the test to her. It consisted primarily of sticking needles into her arms and legs. Pat hated needles but agreed to have the EMG the following week.

The next day, her sister noticed that Pat was walking funny, almost as if she was a little tipsy, but Pat never drank alcohol.

The sister called Onslow, who referred her back to Lyons, who told her to call Baker: trouble with walking is a neurologist's territory.

Baker instructed her to have Pat come in sooner for the EMG.

That night, Pat's speech started to slur. She also seemed to be confused. She didn't know where she was or what she was doing. She'd watch television and not be able to tell her sister what she had seen.

Once again, her sister made the rounds on the telephone: Onslow to Lyons to Baker.

Baker said he'd see them the next afternoon in his office.

Pat's sister didn't think they could wait that long. She brought Pat to the hospital, and Pat was once again admitted, onto Dr. Onslow's service.

Onslow saw her at seven-thirty in the morning, just before he was scheduled to perform his first operation of the day, another partial gastric resection on a patient with morbid obesity.

Pat did not recognize him. In fact, she had no idea where she was.

She told him she hadn't vomited in weeks. And she told him all about the wonderful meal she'd eaten the night before, describing it in detail: steak and potatoes, salad with blue cheese dressing, and chocolate cream pie.

"What did Onslow do?" I asked Jeff.

"He ordered a few routine lab tests, gave her some IV fluids—dextrose and water—and went off to surgery."

"No vitamins?" I asked, already anticipating the answer. Jeff was a malpractice lawyer, and this was the story of a client of his.

"No."

"Thiamine?" I suggested weakly, hoping for Pat Seerey's sake that it had been ordered, for by this time the diagnosis was obvious: Pat Seerey had been starving. She undoubtedly did not look like a victim of starvation, for she was still overweight, but she been morbidly obese to start with.

She'd been starving for many months, having taken in no food (the meal she'd described to Onslow had been a confabulation)—no calories, no proteins, no fats, no carbohydrates, and no vitamins.

That final element was the culprit. The lack of vitamins—vitamin deficiency—can easily destroy the nervous system, both the peripheral nerves and the brain.

Pat had evidence of neuropathy—tingling of her feet—as well as something going wrong inside her brain—imbalance, confusion, and memory loss. Anyone could tell that.

"Thiamine?" I repeated halfheartedly.

"Now why would he want to do that?" Jeff replied sarcastically.

So much for Jack Onslow, general surgeon. He'd missed the diagnosis and, more important, he'd neglected to treat her at a time when treatment might well have saved her brain.

At one-thirty, Lyons saw her. Pat still didn't know where she was until Lyons suggested that it was a hotel, and then she remembered having made her reservations. She thought she knew him but said his name was Faber. Red Faber. She also thought it was 1948.

Lyons asked her if she had been vomiting.

Of course not.

Was she eating?

Yes.

Had she had lunch?

Of course.

What?

Soup, salad, macaroni and cheese, and ice cream. She'd eaten every morsel.

Lyons nodded and then ordered some liver function tests, changed the IV fluid to saline, and requested that Baker see her in consultation.

"Vitamins?" I asked Jeff again.

"No."

"Thiamine?" I persisted. It was thiamine deficiency that was causing her problem.

"Of course not."

Silly me.

"Was she eating at all?"

"No. According to the nurse's notes, the sister reported that the patient vomited every time she ate anything. They also noted that she'd refused both breakfast and lunch."

Baker came by at six o'clock, right after he finished seeing patients in his office.

Pat had no idea who he was.

That wasn't so strange; she had only seen him once in her life, and for a brief visit.

Did her feet still burn?

No.

She thought she was in a hotel. A man named Red Faber was with her.

Baker asked her if she was still vomiting.

Of course not.

Had she had lunch?

Yes.

What?

Meat loaf, gravy, mashed potatoes, salad, cake, and two rolls with butter.

"Vitamins?" I interrupted.

"No. In his note, Baker remarked that her excellent dietary history made any vitamin deficiency unlikely. Especially since her feet were no longer bothering her."

"No thiamine?" I asked once again.

"No thiamine."

"How did he explain the hotel bit? And Red Faber?"

"Her private life was not any of his concern."

"And I suppose she ate no dinner."

"According to the nursing notes, it was sitting there untouched the entire time that Baker was with her. He did order a CAT scan, an EEG, and an EMG."

The story was becoming increasingly painful. Stupidity is always that way, especially stupidity that harms someone else's brain.

The question now was how badly Pat's brain and her life had been damaged.

She'd been admitted on Thursday. It was late Friday when Baker saw her. None of the tests he had ordered could be done until Monday. No one seemed to mind; none of the tests had been ordered on an emergency basis.

Over the weekend, Pat continued to vomit from time to time and eat practically nothing.

The progression of her neurologic disease was all nicely documented in the nursing notes. On Saturday, Pat stopped talking to the nurse except to say "yes" or "no," and her answers seemed to have no logical relationship to their questions. Late Sunday night, she stopped talking altogether. By Monday morning, she was in coma.

Onslow saw her at seven-thirty. He was due in the operating room at eight-thirty.

He had no idea what to do for coma. Coma isn't a surgical problem. He signed off the case and transferred her to Lyons.

Lyons saw her at nine-thirty. Coma is a neurologic problem, so Lyons paged Baker. Baker was at his office. He suggested that they call the neurosurgeon, Glen Moulder.

Moulder was in the hospital and he came right down to see Pat. He had no idea what had happened to her, but he knew what tests to order: CAT scan, STAT, angiogram. He administered them himself; they were all normal.

There was nothing that required an operation. No neurosurgery meant no need for a neurosurgeon. He signed off.

Baker arrived and examined Pat.

"He found nystagmus," I ventured, always the optimist.

"What's that?" Jeff asked.

He had given me such a complete, documented history that I forgot that he wasn't a neurology resident but a lawyer.

"Jerky eye movements."

"Right."

"So he gave her thiamine."

"Wrong. He ordered an EEG. He thought that the jerky eye movements were part of a seizure. So he ordered a STAT EEG."

"And it showed no seizure activity."

"Correct."

"Just severe, generalized slowing."

"Right again."

"What did he do next?"

"A spinal tap."

"Which was normal."

"Not quite."

"It contained a few white cells," I guessed.

"Yes."

"So he made a diagnosis of viral encephalitis."

"That's what the man did."

"When did she get her thiamine?"

"About four days later. She was still in a coma, and they moved her from the surgical unit to a medical floor."

"Who ordered the thiamine?"

"The medical student who was working as an extern."

"Why?"

"He always gives vitamins to patients who have been on IVs for a week. He was taught that during the second year of medical school."

Over the next few days, Pat Seerey woke up, but she never returned to normal. The incidents in the hospital had occurred twenty-three months before Jeff's phone call.

The significance of that time lag was not lost on me. In Illinois, there is a statute of limitations. A malpractice suit must be filed within twenty-four months of the event.

To prove malpractice, two criteria must be fulfilled;

1. The physician, a hospital, or someone else who is responsible for a patient must have "deviated from the standard of care." He or she or its agents must have done something they shouldn't have or neglected to do something they should have done. In essence, there must have been an act of negligence.

2. That deviation or act of negligence must have done harm to the patient.

If a doctor screws up right and left and the patient isn't harmed, then there can be no damages. Such suits rarely come up. Patients who have not been injured or who do not believe they've been injured rarely seek out malpractice attorneys. Conversely, if the doctor does nothing wrong but something bad happens to the patient, there is no malpractice, but the patient may well find a lawyer who will file suit.

With respect to the Pat Seerey case, the first question was already answered in my mind. The doctors had erred, but had they done any permanent harm to the once-fat young woman?

Jeff described her present condition. She could not walk without assistance. She could talk but she couldn't remember much of anything that was new. She remembered almost everything up to about the time of her surgery. Since then, nothing. She couldn't even remember if she ate breakfast, must less what she ate.

Damage had been to done to her. Had they given her thiamine on time, the damage would have been avoided. And any one of them could have done it; they all had the chance.

Pat had a disease named after two physicians who never met. One was a German neurologist, the other a Russian psychiatrist: Carl Wernicke and Sergei Korsakoff. They were contemporaries. Wernicke lived from 1848 to 1905 and Korsakoff from 1854 to 1900. Wernicke held various chairs in neurology in Germany and described a condition we now call ''Wernicke's encephalopathy''—an acute neurologic disorder with three characteristic components:

1. Gait imbalance
2. Altered mentation
3. Jerky eye movements known as nystagmus

Pat had developed all three problems. Her sister had been aware of Pat's drunken gait and had told the doctors about it. Pat's mental changes should have been obvious to even the most casual observer. Baker had been the only one to look at her eyes and see the jerky eye movements.

Korsakoff worked in Moscow and was the first physician to recognize a peculiar mental disorder in alcoholic patients who also had peripheral neuropathy—injury to the nerves as they go out of the nervous system itself to travel to their destinations in the rest of the body. The neuropathy was due to the vitamin deficiencies caused by the patient's alcoholism. The commonest symptom of such neuropathies is a feeling of numbness, tingling, or burning in the feet.

Pat's problem started out with burning feet. Frank Baker realized that she had a peripheral neuropathy, which was why he ordered an EMG. That test is designed to give us information on the function of the nerves as they course throughout the body.

The mental disorder that Korsakoff observed is now called Korsakoff's psychosis. Korsakoff described it in these words:

At times it appears in the form of sharply delineated weakness of the mental sphere, at times in the form of confusion with characteristic mistakes in orientation for place, time and situation and at times as an almost pure form of acute amnesia where the recent memory is most severely involved while the remote memory is well preserved . . . Some have suffered so widespread a memory loss that they literally forget everything immediately.

In a series of carefully written papers, Korsakoff defined the major characteristics of "his" psychosis:

1. Disorientation to time. Pat thought it was 1948.
2. Disorientation to place and situation. She thought she was in a hotel with Red Faber, whoever he was.
3. Amnesia. She couldn't remember her doctors or that she hadn't eaten her meals or that she had been vomiting or where she was.
4. An inability to lay down new memories. Had she eaten lunch? She had no memory of the actual event.
5. Confabulation. She made up answers: she couldn't recall lunch, so she described a meal, and her doctors believed her.

Pat had all the components of Wernicke's encephalopathy, as well as the manifestations of Korsakoff's psychosis. While Wernicke and Korsakoff originally described their disorders as separate entities, the research of subsequent neurologists, especially two Americans who worked together, Raymond D. Adams and Maurice Victor, has shown that these syndromes are two aspects of the same disease, a disease we now call Wernicke-Korsakoff syndrome. The pathology of both is identical. So is the cause—thiamine deficiency.

Thiamine is a vitamin, and it works the way all vitamins work, by functioning as a coenzyme. All life depends upon enzymes, proteins that carry out a specific biochemical reaction. Glucose, the brain's major source of energy, must be broken down or metabolized before it can be used. Each step in this metabolic process is carried out by a specific protein or enzyme. The enzyme must be coupled with a vitamin, and if the vitamin is deficient, the enzyme simply doesn't work.

If thiamine is absent, those enzymes that require thiamine stop functioning.

As a result, glucose metabolism comes to a standstill, and because the brain depends on glucose metabolism, the brain cells are forced to turn to other sources of energy. Brain cells are programmed to keep functioning, and if they can't use glucose, all that is left is their own constituents, the fats that make up the cells themselves.

To maintain function, the cells begin to metabolize themselves. They sacrifice structure to maintain function.

Then function fails, and the cells metabolize themselves to death.

Brain damage.

Pat Seerey.

If this happens over a short time, the patient may develop a pure Wernicke's encephalopathy. If it happens over many months or years, a pure Korsakoff's psychosis may be seen. Most often, it develops in a few months, and the patient has the mixed features of Wernicke-Korsakoff syndrome.

Pat Seerey started with the burning feet of neuropathy ("neuritis") that is due to vitamin deficiency. Then came the imbalance and altered mentation of Wernicke's encephalitis, followed closely by all the components of Korsakoff's psychosis.

The diagnosis was obvious, as was the cause—thiamine deficiency.

As was the relationship of her acute disorder to her present state—she had the memory loss and imbalance characteristic of patients who survive severe Wernicke-Korsakoff syndrome.

"Had there been any malpractice?" Jeff asked me.

"Of course."

"By whom?"

"All of them. Onslow should have known that gastric resections can cause vitamin deficiencies that can result in severe neurologic problems."

"But he's a surgeon, not a neurologist," Jeff protested, playing devil's advocate.

"It's his business to know the complications of his procedure. Besides, many relevant cases have been published in the surgical journals. Surgeons are supposed to read those journals. She was losing weight at a horrendous pace and vomiting. She should have been getting vitamins as soon as she started vomiting."

"He gave her a prescription for multivitamin capsules. Extra strength."

"Not a prescription for capsules—whatever the strength. Shots. She was vomiting daily. Onslow's in."

"Who else?"

"Lyons. He referred her for surgery and continued to follow her. It's his business to know the complications."

"Lyons is in, then," Jeff agreed.

"Baker as well. He should have made a diagnosis of vitamin-deficiency neuropathy and started treatment the first time he saw her. He also should have made a diagnosis of Wernicke-Korsakoff syndrome as soon as he saw her in the hospital."

"Baker disagrees. He says Wernicke's syndrome occurs only in alcoholics. He says he doesn't even consider that diagnosis unless a patient is an alcoholic."

"Bull," I replied articulately. "It was described in nonalcoholics who had persistent vomiting long ago. Every neurologist knows that."

"How long ago?"

"1877."

"By whom?"

"Wernicke. In his first patient. She was a young woman who drank sulfuric acid in an attempt to commit suicide and screwed up her stomach and esophagus. Every time she tried to eat, she vomited. Just like Pat Seerey," I editorialized.

Was I willing to testify against these physicians?

I was willing. I would not be testifying against physicians, but on behalf of Pat Seerey. And she deserved her day in court.

Pat never got her day in court. The case was settled without a trial. She was awarded more than two million dollars but, of course, she can't remember how much money she received or why.

She thinks it's 1967.

She only recognizes people she met before the surgery.

She has no idea who Jeff Wright is or what he does for a living. Or who I am. Or who Jack Onslow is.

But she is down to 141 pounds—not counting her wheelchair.

Author's Note

The neurologic complications of gastric surgery for morbid obesity have been described only in medical literature. The most recent compilation is: J. M. Abarbanel et al., "Neurologic Complications after Gastric Restriction Surgery for Morbid Obesity," *Neurology* 37 (1987): 196–200.

An English translation of Korsakoff's original paper is available: M. Victor and P. I. Yakovlev, "S. S. Korsakoff's Psychic Disorder in Conjunction with Peripheral Neuritis," *Neurology* 5 (1955): 394–406.

=21=

Neurologic Apocrypha

No doubt by disease of some part of the brain the deaf mute might lose his natural system of signs which are of some speech value to him.
—Hughlings Jackson, 1878

The books of the Bible are accepted as such either because they were written by God (the Five Books of Moses) or written by prophets inspired by God. Other ancient Hebrew writings of similar vintage, such as Maccabees I and Maccabees II, although of great significance, have not been so canonized and are considered to be "apocryphal"—not quite to have made the grade. Important, but not fully accepted as part of the revealed truth.

The steps that are required for a "new" neurologic disorder to become recognized as part of the "canon" of neurologic diseases are just as rigorous and just as well codified as are the rules for the Bible. First, the afflicted patient must have been seen and examined during his or her life by a neurologist. This may not seem to be a stringent qualification, but at the end of World War II, there were only a few hundred neurologists in the United States, and even today, there are fewer than 300 neurologists in the United Kingdom (a ratio of one neurologist per 150,000 people). Obviously, in such situations many individuals with neurologic problems escape the scrutiny of a neurologist. Second, the patient must die, preferably of the disease itself. The reason for this requirement is obvious if you think about it. In the days before modern imaging techniques (CAT scans, MRI scans), the only way to be certain that a set of neurologic signs and symptoms was due to an injury of a specific area of the brain was to do an autopsy, to study the brain, and to correlate the findings of the autopsy with the results of detailed neurologic examinations performed during life.

One advantage of this rigorous system is apparent. Guesswork is eliminated. But there are also disadvantages or limitations:

1. All neurologic problems are not uniformly fatal; thus, some patients with "interesting" problems may not die of their disease.
2. Not all who die undergo autopsies.

Ever since I began writing for the nonmedical public, I have been receiving letters from patients whose medical evaluation will never be complete enough to become part of the neurologic canon, yet whose disorders add something to our understanding of the brain and its function. These are the stories that make up the neurologic apocrypha.

Mrs. Weinstein was fifty-seven when she wrote to me. She had read my first novel, *Sins of Commission* and had enjoyed the book, but that was not why shy had written. This was not fan mail.

"I have migraine headaches," she explained.

She had been dealing with her migraine headaches for some forty-five years. She knew what to do when she had one of them. They were part of her life, not something for which she continued to seek medical advice. In fact, they had been less of a problem during the past ten years than they had been for the previous thirty-five years.

Did she really have true migraines? I wondered. In popular usage, the term *migraine* is used to refer to any severe or "sick" headache. Medically speaking, that is not correct. Migraine headaches are headaches in which the pain is related to the sudden, severe stretching of blood vessels to the head or brain. Because of the mechanism involved (stretching or dilation of the arteries), the pain invariably has a throbbing component. This throbbing is due to further dilation of the tender arteries as the heart pumps blood into them.

Mrs. Weinstein went on to describe her headaches—flashing lights followed by a throbbing pain associated with nausea. She had migraines.

"I am writing you because of a mistake that Paul Richardson made on page 263 of *Sins of Commission*.

Paul Richardson was the neurologist/protagonist of the novel.

I immediately reached up to my shelf and pulled down a copy of the book. The sequence she was referring to was one of his teaching sessions, the subject of which was migraine headaches. What else?

As always, Paul Richardson began his teaching rounds with a question:

"Tell me what sorts of things can cause migraine headaches."

"Foods," the student replied.

"What kinds of foods?"

"Cheese."

"Do you know what kind?"

Silence.

"Stilton and Camembert," Paul explained. "Especially the rind of Camembert. But do you know why these cheeses cause headaches?" Richardson continued without giving the students or residents a chance to respond, to be right or wrong. "All the authorities say it's because these foods contain something that directly acts on the blood vessels, a chemical called tyramine. Tyramine causes sudden dilation of selected arteries according to most migraine specialists and this elicits a migraine headache. That's what everybody says. But do you know what food contains the highest amount of tyramine?"

Silence. A silence that Richardson finally understood meant, Slow down. Teach. Don't lecture. Give them a chance. Do it right. He turned to his senior resident.

"Pickled herring," the resident replied.

"Absolutely correct, and there's never been a case of pickled herring causing a migraine."

Enough of Paul Richardson.

I turned back to Mrs. Weinstein's letter. What was it that she was trying to tell me?

"I guess," the letter continued, "I am the exception that proves the rule. Other than MSG, pickled herring is the only food that would cause migraine in me within a half hour. I had suffered with migraine around my menstrual cycle from the age of ten until I reached menopause. However, it did not matter at what time of the month I ate foods containing MSG and pickled herring to get a headache. I was a lover of herring, so I did not give it up without experimenting to see if it would cause a headache. Even a half teaspoon of pickled herring, chopped, caused a headache.

"Presently, I am not getting migraine headaches but I'm afraid to try herring again, so severe were the headaches it caused. I would appreciate your comments."

As soon as I read her letter, I called Mrs. Weinstein. We talked for forty minutes, and at the end of our conversation I did not know very much more than I did before I had called her.

She did have migraine headaches, and in fact, she had what are now classified as "classic" migraines. Classic migraines have two phases. In the first, the patient has symptoms other than headache. These symptoms are thought to be due to the sudden constriction or clamping down of selected blood vessels. Mrs. Weinstein's premonitory symptoms or "aura" (warning) consisted of irregular flashing lights off to one side. This is the commonest of the classic auras. After ten to fifteen minutes, the visual sensation gradually disappears, and the headache itself starts as a severe throbbing pain on one side of the head or the other.

Mrs. Weinstein's migraines had started at about the time of menarche and had decreased since menopause, a common but incompletely understood phenomenon.

And they were precipitated each time she ate pickled herring. And oh, how she loved pickled herring! She had tried every brand she could find to see if one was safer than the others, but they all caused her to have migraines.

She was truly a first and, I would be willing to wager, the first patient in the world in whom pickled herring caused migraines. Paul Richardson, of course, had not made up the story about no patient ever before having reported this sequence. It was pointed out by one of the world's experts on migraine, George W. Bruyn of the University of Leiden. I had to tell George about Mrs. Weinstein, and not just George, but the entire world of migraine specialists, as well. The ever-elusive pickled herring headache had been found. Without it, the notion that tyramine in foods was the chemical factor that triggered migraines was on shaky ground. I did not realize how difficult it would be for such an apocryphal tale to be canonized.

Since I had never examined the patient, I felt that a brief letter to the editor of an appropriate journal was the best approach, and wrote to *Clinical Neuropharmacology*. That was where George Bruyn had pointed out the dearth of pickled herring headaches. (I chose to have Paul Richardson act as author of this letter since it was Paul who had stimulated the patient to write to me in the first place, and besides, I felt he deserved to make an appearance in the accepted medical literature.)

In due time, the following letter was received by the editor-in-chief of *Clinical Neuropharmacology:*

To the editor:

In his review of the biochemical basis of migraine, Bruyn cast doubt on the role of tyramine in precipitation of migraine headaches (1). According to Bruyn, the tyramine load present in marinated herring is much larger than that used to precipitate migraine headaches in known migraneurs (2), yet he had treated hundreds of migraneurs and had never seen a patient in whom migraines were induced by this food. I had also previously never been aware of a case of pickled (marinated) herring causing a migraine (3). I have recently, however, discovered such a patient. This woman had read the two vulgarizations of my activities (4,5) and wrote the following letter to me discussing the role of pickled herring in causing her migraine headaches.

From her description, it is clear that pickled (marinated) herring can elicit migraines in at least one susceptible individual. Whether or not this is related to tyramine is unclear. Why this occurred in the United States and not in Holland, where the per capita consumption of herring is much greater, is also unclear. It is possible that the biochemical nature of American pickled herring is not identical to that of Dutch marinated herring.

1. G. W. Bruyn, "The Biochemical Basis of Migraine," *Clinical Neuropharmacology* 1(1977):185–214.
2. E. Hannington, P. E. Mullen, and A. H. Kellow, "Dietary Migraine and Tyramine Metabolism," *Nature* (London) 230(1971):246–248.
3. P. Richardson, (1975): Personal communication, quoted in H. L. Klawans, *Sins of Commission,* (New York: Signet, 1987), p. 264.
4. H. L. Klawans, *Sins of Commission* (New York: Signet, 1987).
5. H. L. Klawans, *Informed Consent* (New York: Signet, 1986).

Sincerely,

Paul Richardson, MD
Professor and Chairman,
Department of Neurology
Austin Flint Medical School

The editor immediately accepted the letter for what it was, a minor but significant contribution to medical knowledge, and passed it on to the publisher for inclusion in the next issue of the journal. The publisher, in a case of blatant censorship, rejected it. Publishers have, I'm afraid, lost their sense of proportion and their sense of humor.

In other correspondence, two readers wrote me about a different neurologic disorder. Both had been reminded of the story by reading my clinical tale about a young woman, a skilled musician, who suddenly lost her ability to play her oboe ("Broca's Amusica" in *Toscanini's Fumble*). The first letter, from Iowa, did not give enough detail to analyze.

I was a student at the University of Iowa, in Iowa City, and took a course in semantics from Wendell Johnson. He discussed briefly the case of an Indian who lost the ability to communicate via sign language. He said that this might be thought of as "asymbolia." No other symptoms were apparent, and he did not discuss any underlying physical basis as you did. This leaves me wondering if the same problems were present.

I could not remember ever having read or heard of a patient who had the isolated problem of the loss of the ability to communicate via sign language. But was that really what had happened to this Indian? The story was now thirdhand, so that its apocryphal position was compounded by its anecdotal nature. Had the patient really just lost the ability to sign and nothing else? This question relates to a far more basic issue of brain function: Is the ability to communicate via sign language truly an isolated function, unassociated with any other abilities? If so, it would mean that signing ability is located in a specific region of the brain that subserves no other function. Had the unique nature of the loss of signing been confirmed by a neurologist? Had the patient died? Was an autopsy done? And besides, which sign language had he used? American Sign Language (ASL) or the sign language used by American Indians for intertribal negotiations?

There was no way for me to get answers to these questions, and to understand the "asymbolia" of this Indian, I needed such answers. Neurologically, the key question is whether "asymbolia" is a form of aphasia or a type of apraxia. Is ASL a true language, managed in the brain like any spoken language, or is it a set of hand symbols controlled by regions of the brain that are not dedicated primarily to communication via the spoken word?

In "Broca's Amusica," I presented a simplified approach to aphasia:

First, aphasia is the loss of the use of language.

Second, aphasia is always due to a lesion of the dominant hemisphere for speech. In right-handed individuals, the dominant hemisphere is always the left hemisphere; in left-handers the left hemisphere still tends to be dominant for speech.

Third, if the patient has more trouble producing words than understanding them, the problem is located toward the front of the dominant hemisphere. The term *Broca's aphasia* or *expressive aphasia* is used to denote an aphasic state in which expression is more involved than comprehension. Patients with Broca's aphasia can understand relatively well. They can follow commands, even complicated ones, but cannot really speak. Their speech consists of a few syllables or words, and they cannot name objects correctly. The right words evade them. Pierre Broca was not the first physician to describe such a patient, but his name became attached to this type of aphasia because he was the first to associate it with a lesion in a specific location of the brain, namely, the third frontal convolution on the left, a location now known as Broca's area.

Fourth, if patients can produce speech fluently but cannot understand what is said to them and cannot follow commands, they have a lesion farther back in their brains. This lesion is called *receptive aphasia* or *Wernicke's aphasia,* named after Carl Wernicke, who did for receptive aphasia what Broca did for expressive aphasia. (Wernicke made other contributions to neurology. His role in describing the Wernicke-Korsakoff syndrome is discussed in chapter 20, "Morbid Obesity.")

And fifth, all the rest is mere commentary. Neurologists have described many minor variations of these speech disorders. These subtle differences make no difference to most of us or to most of our patients.

Given these guidelines for aphasia, wouldn't asymbolia be considered a form of aphasia? Not necessarily, for it could be a type of apraxia.

But what precisely is apraxia? It has been traditional in neurology to quote the early neurologist Dejeune, who pointed out that it is far easier to define what apraxia is not than to say exactly what it is. Apraxia is the inability to perform a learned motor act in the absence of any other specific type of neurologic defect that would prevent the performance of that act. Apraxic patients are awake and alert. They understand what the act is. They are not weak or paralyzed, nor is their motor system disrupted by abnormal movements or the inability to coordinate or synergise movements.

An example might be a patient who can follow all other simple commands, and therefore understands, but who cannot stick out his tongue when asked to do so. Yet he unconsciously licks his lips with his tongue, demonstrating that his tongue movement itself is normal. Hence apraxia for tongue movement.

So is asymbolia an aphasia or an apraxia?

What difference would it make?

To the patient, very little; to neurologists and other students of brain function, it's an interesting problem. If the loss of the ability to communicate via ASL is an aphasia, then ASL—a nonverbal (nonspoken) language—is learned and controlled by the dominant hemisphere for speech, the left hemisphere. If the loss of ASL is an apraxia unassociated with any aphasia, then this nonverbal language may well be controlled by the right or nondominant hemisphere. After all, most apraxias for complex movements are caused by disorders of the nondominant side of the brain.

I went to the library to look for an answer but couldn't find very much to satisfy me. MacDonald Critchley, the neurologic world's preeminent authority on the parietal lobes (the seat of most apraxias), wrote an article titled "Aphasia in a Partial Deaf Mute" in 1937. The patient he described gradually lost his hearing beginning at age 7 and was totally deaf by age

14. At age 42 he had a stroke with a right-sided paralysis and lost what little articulated speech he had retained over the years, as well as his ability to read lips or sign language and to sign with either hand.

The interpretation of this patient's problem was obvious: He had three neurologic disorders:

1. Right-sided weakness.
2. Aphasia.
3. Loss of signing.

The first two disorders pointed to the left hemisphere; the third had to have its basis on that same side. In Critchley's patient, the loss of signing was an aphasia, but one question still remained unanswered. If he had learned signing as his primary language, would it still have been localized in the dominant hemisphere if it were not true language, but a motor skill?

More recently, neurologists have had the opportunity to study one other such patient, a twenty-seven-year-old woman with normal speech and hearing, who had a master's degree in rehabilitation of the deaf and who had learned ASL as an adult and used it every day of her life. She also had epilepsy that could not be controlled by anticonvulsant medications. Her seizures appeared to come from her right temporal lobe, and her neurologist (Antinio Damasio and his associates from the University of Iowa) studied her to see if she might be a candidate for surgery for her epilepsy.

If her left hemisphere was dominant for language, then surgery on the right side of her brain would not disrupt her linguistic abilities. Aphasia, after all, is due to a lesion of the dominant (left) hemisphere.

But what about signing? If it is a spoken language, it would also be on the dominant hemisphere. But is it? Sign language depends upon the manipulation of visual-spatial relationships, an ability that is almost always housed in the nondominant hemisphere of hearing individuals. If her signing ability was truly controlled by the nondominant hemisphere, then surgery there would impair it.

Aphasia or apraxia. The same hemisphere for both spoken language and signing? Or opposite ones? It was no longer an idle philosophical issue, but one with major clinical relevance.

But how could it be answered?

By what is called a Wada test. In this procedure, a fast-acting barbiturate is injected directly into one of the carotid arteries. The side of the brain that the artery feeds quickly "goes to sleep," while the other side is spared. If speech is located on the injected side, aphasia should develop.

If it isn't, no aphasia should occur. In this young woman, such as injection could be followed by testing both speech and signing.

And that is just what Damasio and his associates did. In their Wada test, they injected Amytal directly into the patient's left carotid artery. She developed aphasia for both English (as a spoken, verbal language) and ASL. The surgery therefore, would not cause either aphasia or the loss of ASL skills. She underwent the operation, a partial removal of her right temporal lobe, and suffered neither aphasia nor any difficulty with ASL. Thus, the loss of ASL is an aphasia, but can it ever occur without any other evidence of aphasia?

The patient mentioned briefly in the reader's letter suggested that that could happen. The impairment of ASL that Damasio and his associates had observed during the Wada test had lasted longer than the drug-induced aphasia. This finding suggests that while aphasia and loss of signing may be related, they might occur independently—that there can be a loss of signing without aphasia. This situation was observed for several minutes as part of a Wada test. Had it ever happened to a patient?

The second letter gave me the answer. It described a patient in far more detail. He was a right-handed hearing individual who learned ASL to communicate with a much younger deaf brother. The patient developed rheumatic heart disease but had no neurologic problems until he was thirty-eight and suddenly lost the ability to sign. His ability to speak and understand was normal, but he could not sign at all, and his right hand was clumsy, (that symptom only lasted a week or two).

The clumsiness of the right hand clinched it. The lesion—a stroke that was most likely due to an embolus caused by his rheumatic heart disease—had to be in his left hemisphere. Therefore, his loss of signing without aphasia for spoken language was due to a disease of that same hemisphere. It could happen: "asymbolia without aphasia," it was a publishable case, and all that was needed was a CAT scan to demonstrate the exact location of the stroke and an examination of the patient.

I read on. The patient died two years later of his rheumatic heart disease.

In people who have learned a verbal language, ASL is controlled by the dominant hemisphere (for speech). Is this also the case in completely non-verbal individuals? We don't know, but the existence of a separate location on the dominant hemisphere for signing makes me suspect that it is.

Just one more bit of apocrypha. No journal publishes articles without proof. As a result, neurologists still wonder if asymbolia can occur without aphasia.

It can. And it already has. Damasio's case study showed that it could happen in a chemically induced alteration in brain function, not that it had ever happened in a naturally occurring disease. Only the patient described to me in a letter from a reader did that. That letter was not written by a neurologist, nor was it sent to a neurological journal. And there had never been a detailed neurological examination or a CAT scan or an autopsy. No data, no published medical truth, but the truth nonetheless. Medically we did not "know" that aphasia and control of the dominant hand were two functions that went together until the latter half of the nineteenth century. But that association had been observed more than two thousand years earlier during the Babylonian exile, canonized in the Bible, and been repeated daily as part of a Jewish prayer: "If I forget Thee, O Jerusalem, let my right hand lose its cunning. . . . let my tongue cleave to the roof of my mouth." A perfect description of Broca's aphasia associated with paralysis of the dominant right hand. And it's not quoted in a single neurological textbook.

Author's Note

The article by Antonio Damasio et al., "Sign Language Aphasia during Left Hemisphere Amytal Injection" is in *Nature* (232[1987]:363–65), while one by MacDonald Critchley appeared in *Brain* (61[1937]:163–69). Critchley's book, *Silent Language* (London: Bullerworth, 1975), is a thorough exploration of all nonverbal forms of communication and is recommended to all. It covers subjects ranging from gestures to pantomime to sign languages and Asian dances. It is hard to find, but well worth the effort. Incidentally, I am the editor in chief of *Clinical Neuropharmacology*.

My Mother's Clinic:
The Triad of Steele, Richardson,
and Olszewski

Two of the most difficult tasks a writer can undertake, to write the truth about himself and about his mother.

—Frank O'Connor

It was a typical Thursday afternoon—my time at the Parkinson Disease Clinic. In five hours, I would see twenty patients—four new patients whom I had never met and sixteen others who would come for follow-up visits, to have their disease and its treatment evaluated and the treatment altered, if necessary. Fortunately, I did not have to do all this by myself. I had two first-year neurology residents, one senior neurology resident, and my mother to help me. The residents would evaluate some of the patients first, especially the new patients, and then we would see them together and discuss them. That process occasionally even saved time.

It was my mother who really made it all succeed. In many ways, she *was* the Parkinson Disease Clinic. She greeted the patients personally and talked to them individually. The patients would often come early—sometimes even an hour or more before their scheduled appointments—to have time to speak to her, to drink a cup of her fresh-brewed coffee, to eat one or two of her homemade cookies, but especially to visit with her. That created a space problem, for the waiting room was not large enough to accommodate all the patients and their spouses or "significant others" at one time. It also created another problem—no one wanted to be seen first. It wouldn't be right to take up space in the waiting room after they'd been seen by their doctor.

Getting my mom to work in the clinic had not been easy. She'd completed nursing training and had been working as a nurse when she met my father, who was doing his internship at the same hospital. But she had not practiced in almost forty years and had no interest in doing so. In 1968, my father died, and I tried to figure out a way to get my mother back on track. Having her take charge of the clinic seemed to be the best bet. She loved working with people and could organize anything. She'd been president of more women's groups than I could remember. And now she was nearing seventy, and leadership in these groups had passed on to the next generation. All that was left were bridge clubs or mah-jongg groups.

Had she been born forty or fifty years later, she would have gotten her MBA and been a successful career woman. But she had been born in 1900, so she took her degree in nursing, married, and raised her family.

I told her what I wanted her to do.

No soap. She wasn't interested. She hadn't done any nursing in forty years. She didn't remember any of it, and besides she hadn't tried to keep up. She wasn't going to make a fool of herself.

It wasn't nursing, I explained. It was administration and . . .

"And what?" she demanded.

"Humanizing the clinic—giving it a personal touch. Making the patients feel welcome."

It almost worked. She was wavering. Then I remembered a story that I hadn't thought about in years. When she was in training, one of her friends died in a diabetic coma just two weeks before the first shipment of insulin arrived in Chicago. Had that nursing student gone into a coma two weeks later, she might well have lived forty more years. It was a story my mother had told me more than once. Its moral had long been part of her approach to life.

"And Mom," I said, "I have the insulin these people need." It was not far from the truth. Many diabetics are diabetic because their bodies cannot make insulin. Without insulin to treat them, their future would be bleak, at best. Patients with Parkinson's disease (PD) cannot manufacture dopamine in the brain, and without this substance, their disease progresses inexorably. L-dopa might be considered the insulin we give to diabetics. It replaces the missing chemical. Once given in PD L-dopa enters the brain, where it is transformed into the missing dopamine.

"I have the insulin, this time," I reiterated.

A tear came into her eye.

"She was my best friend."

I hadn't known that.

"I owe it to her."

She was an immediate success. It wasn't the coffee or the cookies, although they were wonderful, and no matter how many she baked, they all were eaten. It was her. Patients would shuffle in, especially new patients who came to see if they could get this miracle treatment. After she'd talked to them a while, they began getting better. They would stand straighter and shuffle less as they walked from the reception room to an examining room. I don't know what she said. Whatever it was, she gave them the hope and confidence they needed.

Once or twice each Thursday afternoon, my mother would personally bring the patient and the chart into my office, or if one of the residents saw the patient first, she would write brief notes on the charts. Her messages were always succinct: My mother had severe arthritis of her hands. They were always important, containing information that patients or their significant others had shared with her and that she wanted to be sure I didn't miss in my brief interview. Or information patients preferred to share first with her. Or a clinical observation she had made. Examples of her messages abound in my memory:

> Too much dopa?
> Grimaces at meals (wife).
> Patient unaware.
> Mom

> Lost her urine twice.
> Very embarrassed.
> Be gentle.
> Refer to urologist?
> Mom

She made such diagnostic observations, once or twice a month. I won't reveal her batting average, but if she'd batted clean up for the White Sox, the Yankees would have taken fewer pennants away from us.

It was getting late on that particular Thursday afternoon, and it was time for my last patient: sixteen returns seen, three new patients completed. All three would be started on L-dopa. One new patient to go. My mother brought the patient in, with a note on his chart:

Eyes look different.
Not PD.
I'm going home.
Love,
Mom

I looked at the rest of the information on the chart:

Name: Wambsgans
Date of Birth: 1911
(that made him fifty-eight years old).
Reason for referral: L-dopa.

At that time, I was the only neurologist in Chicago who was accepting PD patients for treatment with L-dopa. Mr. Wambsgans had been referred by the United Parkinson Foundation, one of the major national charities involved with PD. Among their services is the referral of patients to physicians with expertise in PD. That did not mean that Mr. Wambsgans had PD, but merely that he had contacted them asking where he could go for L-dopa, and they had referred him to me.

Below this there was another note from my mother: "Diagnosed as PD at Mayo Clinic."

Mr. Wambsgans wobbled into my office. Mom was right: His eyes were all wrong. His upper lids were slightly retracted, so his eyes looked far more prominent than normal, and they never moved. His head was erect, and his eyes were frozen as if focused on the wall above me.

I introduced myself and asked him to sit down. Without turning his head, he rotated his entire body a few degrees, as if he had been carved out of granite, and took a step backwards.

"You are right in front of the chair," I informed him.

"Thank you," he said, and with that, dropped directly into the chair, bounced once, and then slumped toward the right, stopping when his arm hit the arm of the chair.

In a moment, he recovered and straightened himself a bit so he was listing no more than 10 or 12 degrees to his right. His head was still perfectly aligned so that his entire spine was straight as an arrow, an arrow that should have been shot in perpendicular to the seat of the chair but had missed. He sat directly opposite me and stared fixedly at the art above my bookcase. I, too, liked that picture, a small etching by Jacques Villon. But he was there to see me, not to admire my taste in etchings.

Chalk one up for my mother, I said to myself. *Mom 1, Mayo 0.* Of course, my job wasn't done yet. What he didn't have was not the question. The problem was to discover what he did have.

It wasn't only his eyes that showed me he didn't have PD; it was his neck, as well. He sat immobile, like an off-kilter wax statue of Charles de Gaulle. Patients with PD never look like Charles de Gaulle. The rigidity that is basic to their disease increases the tone of all their muscles, including the muscles that are responsible for the maintenance of posture. And this increase in tone is not uniform in all muscles of the body. That's the key—the inequality of parkinsonian rigidity. This inequality always follows the same pattern. It involves flexor muscles more than extensors. A flexor is a muscle that when contracted, *closes* the joint it moves. An extensor, in contrast, *opens* the joint it moves. In PD, flexor tone is greater than extensor tone, and, therefore, the joints tend to be slightly closed. The typical posture of every patient with PD reflects this. The spine is bent forward with the back rounded; the posture is stooped. The hips and knees are bent, as are the elbows. And the neck is invariably tipped forward. The overall posture is reminiscent of a monkey's far more than of Charles de Gaulle's and is thus often called a Simian posture.

So what did Mr. Wambsgans have?

Once again, the first hint came from his neck. He was not just Charles de Gaulle, he was de Gaulle overexaggerated. His neck was not just erect, but extended more than normal. That made his neck tone the opposite of what is normally seen in PD, but typical of another illness. The three physicians who first described Mr. Wambsgans's disorder and who have become an eponym were Steele, Richardson, and Olszewski. The disease also goes by two other names: progressive supranuclear palsy (PSP) and multisystem disease.

Although the last is the easiest to say, it conveys the least information, and because of that has never really caught on. PSP, as it is usually called by those who prefer acronyms to eponyms, shares many features with PD:

1. Increased muscle tone (rigidity), although the distribution of the increased tone is not identical in the two diseases.
2. A slowness of movement. Mr. Wambsgans moved slowly, as if cut from a block of stone, the statue from *Don Giovanni* come to life.
3. Poor balance, with an inability to adjust to threats to posture, resulting in frequent falls. Mr. Wambsgans had fallen into my chair.

The similarities are what had misled the neurologist at the Mayo Clinic. The fact that these similarities exist is not surprising. A single system— the dopamine-producing cells of the substantia nigra—degenerates in PD.

That same system is one of the many that degenerates in PSP. But it is the deterioration of other systems that causes the symptoms that are not ever seen in PD. Three of these symptoms are the keys to making the diagnosis of PSP—the triad that, when present, make the clinical diagnosis of PSP:

1. Hyperextension of the neck (de Gaulle gone overboard.)
2. Abnormal eye movements.
3. Marked difficulty speaking and swallowing.

My mother had been right. It would be the eyes that would make the diagnosis. The eyes are the most distinctive clinical feature of PSP.

> Eyes look wrong.
> Not PD.
>   Mom

I had never seen a patient with PSP before, and was so anxious to examine Mr. Wambsgans's eyes that I didn't even listen to his history. I leaped out from behind my desk and stood directly in front of him.

"Watch my finger," I said.

"Yeth," he lisped at me, his eyes wide open and staring straight at my right forefinger, which I was holding directly in front of him.

I raised my finger up six inches.

His eyes remained frozen in place, not moving as much as a single millimeter.

I tried it again and was met with the same lack of response.

I repeated my instruction; he repeated his slurred reply.

This time, I moved my finger downward. First six, then twelve inches. His eyes never budged.

I repeated my motion, and again his eyes stayed glued in place.

I shifted gears and repeated my instruction. This time I moved my finger laterally. First to the right, then to the left. His response remained the same—no response at all.

I took out my pocket flashlight and held it in front of him, shining it in his eyes and instructing him to follow the light.

Perhaps the light would be an easier target to follow.

Up, down, right, left—nothing.

Time to shift gears again.

"Do what I tell you," I said.

"Yeth, thir."

"Look up."

Nothing happened.

"Look down."

Nothing again.

I repeated my instruction.

No response.

"Look to the right."

"Look to the left."

Direction made no difference.

I gave him other instructions.

"Lift your right hand."

"Put your left hand on your right ear."

These he did, albeit slowly.

I then told him to keep looking forward. I rotated his head to the right. In a normal individual, the eyes remain in the same relative position and aim toward where the head is pointed. His didn't. His eyes stayed where they were, pointed straight at me, and in doing so shifted to his left.

I moved his head to the left.

His eyes shifted to his right, pointing straight at me.

When I moved his head up, the eyes moved down and when I moved his head down, they moved up.

His eyes moved like the eyes of a well-made, expensive children's doll.

Positive doll's-eye movements.

Negative pursuit movements.

Negative voluntary movements.

I had my diagnosis.

PSP.

I impolitely raced out of my office. I had to find someone with whom I could share my discovery. No one was there. The senior resident had left, as had both first-year residents. Even my mother had gone home. The only one who was still in the area who might learn something from my explanation was Mr. Wambsgans. I did my best.

There were, I began, three systems that controlled eye movements: pursuit, voluntary gaze, and doll's eye.

Pursuit refers to eye movements that occur while following an object. Voluntary gaze refers to eye movements directed volitionally by the patient independent of any object in his vision, such as looking to the left when asked to do so. Doll's-eye movements are movements made by the eye within the socket in response to someone else moving the head.

The nerves that produce eye movements are in the base of the brain—the brain stem. The systems that initiate the first two types of movement, pursuit and voluntary gaze, begin in the cerebral hemispheres. Pursuit begins in the occipital lobe, where vision is located. This area sees the object and sends messages to the brain stem to move the eyes to follow it. Voluntary gaze begins in the frontal lobe, where all voluntary movements are organized. The frontal lobe sends messages to the brain stem to initiate voluntary eye movements.

Mr. Wambsgans had neither pursuit nor voluntary gaze. I demonstrated both to him, and though I'm not sure he wanted to go through it again, he was the only audience I had.

The loss of both pursuit and voluntary gaze could mean either of two possibilities:

1. The total loss of all input from above the brain stem nuclei that are responsible for eye movement—a supranuclear palsy—or
2. The inability of the brain stem nuclei themselves to function properly.

Which one was it?

That I knew. He had doll's-eye movements, and their presence depends upon several factors. The brain stem nuclei that control eye movements must be able to respond to an input from the inner ear. This input is generated by movement of the head. But for this input to cause a response, these brain stem nuclei must be free of all control from higher centers. People with normal brains don't have doll's-eye movements precisely because their higher centers prevent such movements.

I had the answer. Mr. Wambsgans had doll's-eye movement, which meant his brain stem was receiving no input from above—which meant he had supranuclear palsy.

Other brain stem nuclei also receive supranuclear inputs, especially those that control speech and swallowing. They, too, are affected in PSP. I already knew that Mr. Wambsgans's speech was involved. I'd heard him slurring his answers to my few questions.

I asked him about swallowing.

He was, he admitted, having problems.

Mr. Wambsgans had all three parts of the triad of Steele, Richardson, and Olszewski.

I took the rest of his history. He had had progressive difficulty for two years. It had started with poor balance and slow movements. He began tripping over objects he somehow didn't see, such as stairs and curbs, even boxes. This is not surprising, considering two of his symptoms—eyes that could not look downward and a head that extended backwards.

I told him what he had.

He'd never heard of PSP, and, furthermore, he wanted only one question answered. Could I help him?

I didn't know.

"Mithuth Klavanth sath you could help me," he said.

Perhaps I could, but, I wasn't that confident. Some of his problems were similar to those of PD; perhaps his symptoms had a similar mechanism, and, if so, perhaps L-dopa would help. It wasn't much; a maybe, two perhaps, and an if, but it was all I had to offer.

I started him on L-dopa, and while it helped a few of those features that were PD-like—his slowness, his balance difficulties, some of his stiffness—it made little practical difference. None of the features of his PSP improved. His neck remained hyperextended and his eyes remained immobile; as a result, he continued to trip. Since he was now able to walk faster, however, he fell harder. Neither his speech nor his swallowing improved.

He came to see me and my mother every month or so and deteriorated before our very eyes. PSP, after all, is just that—progressive. He died about three years after his first visit, of pneumonia.

In 1971, I took a sabbatical of sorts and was away from the clinic for almost three months. My family and I went to Israel, and my mother joined us for the last four weeks. Mr. Wambsgans was one of the patients I saw the first week I got back. By now he was in a wheelchair, and his wife came with him.

"We missed your mother," she said.

"We've all been in Israel," I explained.

"Oh," she replied. "I didn't know you were out of town, too. Did you have a good time?"

I didn't really understand this conversation until Mr. Wambsgans died. My mother was the one who broke the news to me. Mr. Wambsgans had died at home. He'd started to cough and became short of breath and had a high fever. *Pneumonia,* I said to myself. Since there was nothing more we could do for him except prolong his dying, Mrs. Wambsgans decided to keep him at home, but only after discussing the options with my mother. It seems they talked to each other at least once a week.

My mother retired about twelve years after Mr. Wambsgans's first visit to my office. She was over eighty by then, and her arthritis had grown worse. But neither her cookies nor her diagnostic acumen had deteriorated appreciably. I still have one of the last notes she attached to a chart:

Eyes.
Not PD.
M.

She wrote less, since writing was so difficult for her, but she wrote what was needed. Never more and rarely if ever less.

I saw this note before I noticed that my mother had attached it to Katie O'Brien's chart.

Mom had to be wrong this time. Katie O'Brien had PD. She'd had it for fifteen years, and I'd been treating her for it for twelve of those years. She had participted in any number of experimental protocols. She had been patient number 19 on my original L-dopa protocol in 1968—the nineteenth patient I ever placed on L-dopa. And number 17 for Sinemet. Number 11 for bromocriptine. And she had responded to all three.

She had PD. But she was no longer doing well. Of course, she was twelve years older than when I had first treated her, and she'd had her disease for twelve more years. The medicines she'd taken don't cure the disease; they treat the symptoms, and as the disease progresses, there are more and more symptoms to treat. In the years before we had these medications, many patients were bedridden or died after ten to twelve years of the disease.

And so Mrs. O'Brien was worse.

She was much worse than when I had seen her two months before. She stumbled into my office and fell into a chair, with her head erect and her eyes aimed four feet over my head.

Shades of William Wambsgans.

Mom had been right again.

I took a deep breath and got up to examine her eyes.

Pursuit: absent in all directions.

Voluntary gaze: the same.

Doll's-eye movements: present.

PSP.

Mrs. O'Brien no longer just had PD, but that plus something else.

She had PSP.

When had I last tested her eye movements?

I looked through her chart. Two visits earlier—a mere four months before.

Eye movements: normal.
Full range of motion, voluntary and pursuit.

She'd had PD then and was doing fairly well. Her deterioration began one month later. Now she had PSP, and neither the Sinemet nor the bromocriptine were helping much, if at all.

Somehow she retained hope and a confidence that I would be able to help her. Her granddaughter, who'd been about ten when I first saw Mrs. O'Brien, but was now in her twenties, brought her in for her appointments. I mentioned her grandmother's attitude to her one day.

"She wasn't always that way," she began.

That surprised me.

"It was the story your mother told her."

"What story?" I asked.

"When your mother was a nursing student, her best friend died in a diabetic coma just two weeks before the first shipment of insulin arrived in Chicago."

I nodded.

"You can't give up hope. You don't know what may happen in the future. Once you give up hope, you're as good as dead. But I don't have to teach you that."

No, she didn't. My mother already had, long before I became a doctor.

We have changed the natural history of PD. Before L-dopa, it was associated with a significantly decreased life expectancy. Today that is no longer true. Our new medications have added five or more years to the life of the average PD patient. That means an average of five more years for the disease to progress, for more cells to die within the brain.

And for some patients, even more than five years.

And because of this an amazing thing has happened. The natural history of the disease has changed in a few of these patients. PSP and PD used to be entirely separate diseases: A patient either had one or the other. William Wambsgans had PSP; Katie O'Brien had PD.

He did not respond to L-dopa; She did, for ten years. But now she had both diseases; PD plus PSP.

She'd started with PD, and she lived longer than she would have without L-dopa, far longer. Because of that extended life, her disease had progressed. More parts of the brain were involved, and more cells were now dying—cells that did more than just make dopamine, cells that moved the neck, cells that moved the eyes. Now her disease caused new problems, so we gave it a new name: PSP.

And I could not treat the PSP. I couldn't when William Wambsgans got it ten years before and I couldn't when Mrs. O'Brien developed it in 1980. And I still can't.

The fact that this new wrinkle—PSP developing in a patient with PD—was really a testimony to how successfully we had treated her PD was of little consolation to either Mrs. O'Brien or me. The reason that the two diseases were mutually exclusive before the era of L-dopa was because patients died of their PD before they developed PSP.

Mrs. O'Brien's PD responded well to L-dopa; her life was not shortened by PD. She lived on and developed PSP, and in eighteen months she was dead of pneumonia.

PSP used to be rare. I went through an entire residency and never encountered it, and William Wambsgans was the first patient I had ever seen with the disease. Now I see six to eight new PSP patients each year. Most of them are not really "new," however; they are patients like Katie O'Brien who develop PSP after years of PD.

Why?

Is it the fault of the medications?

Any unexpected side effect?

No.

For some unknown reason, selected groups of nerve cells are dying. First those causing PD, and then more slowly and much later, those that result in PSP. You have to survive the first phase for the second phase to occur.

My mother retired in 1982. By 1985, she had progressive angina pectoris, which severely curtailed her activities. Each year, she could do less and less. She never gave up hope. We had an understanding. She would go to her doctor and do whatever he said, but she had decided that she'd wanted to die at home, so I wouldn't admit her to a hospital unless I was sure it would really make a difference.

It was Mr. Wambsgans revisited.

My mother died at home.

After she died, we found boxes of chocolate candy stashed around the apartment, hand-dipped chocolates that she'd ordered and had delivered to her. According to the receipt, she'd gotten her last delivery the day before she'd died.

She wasn't supposed to eat chocolates, but she had one piece each day.

More than once, I'd heard her explain it to my patients. "One cookie a day is good for you. It'll remind you of all the good things you'll be able to do when you get better."

When.

Not "if."

Never "if."

Author's Note

PSP is one of the few neurologic diseases without its own society. Information about this disease is available through the United Parkinson Foundation, 360 West Superior, Chicago, IL 60611.

This is William Wambsgans's second literary appearance. His debut was in my first article, which described my experiences in treating patients with PSP with L-dopa: H. L. Klawans and S. P. Ringel, "Observations on the Efficacy of L-dopa in Progressive Supranuclear Palsy," *European Neurology* 5 (1971): 107–116. When this was written it never occured to me that it would be appropriate to relay information to a nonphysician audience about such a disease and how it affects those who have it.

We discovered one other thing after my mother died. She'd been born in 1899, not 1900. Even in her eighties she never admitted to having been born in the nineteenth century.

ABOUT THE AUTHOR

Harold L. Klawans, M.D., is professor of neurology and pharmacology at
Rush University in Chicago. He is the author of *Toscanini's Fumble* and
The Medicine of History and four novels, *Sins of Commission*, *Informed
Consent*, *The Jerusalem Code*, and *Deadly Medicine* (published in the
United Kingdom).